New cosmetic beauty skincare guide

The expert beauty tips and healthy skin care routine

By

Jennifer D. Elvis

About the author

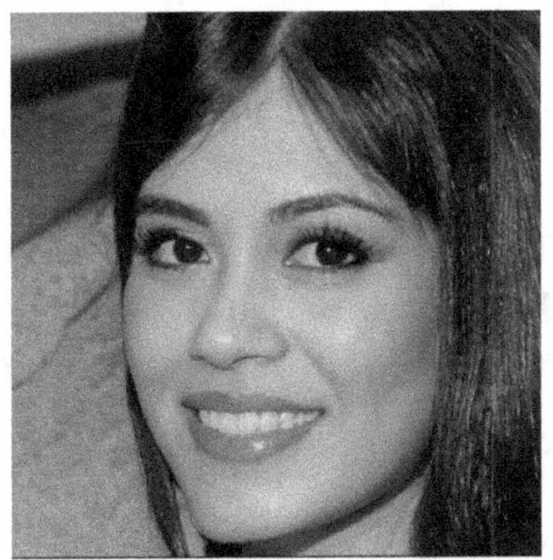

Presenting Jennifer D. Elvis, your confided in a counselor on skincare and cosmetics. Jennifer brings a plenty of skill and experience to the pages of this aide, driven by her adoration for keeping up with shining skin and her significant regard for the magnificence of beauty care products.

Jennifer began her examination of the restorative excellence industry on an individual level. Because she wanted to learn more about the intricacies of skincare and improve her own beauty routine, she immersed herself in the extensive and ever-changing world of beauty practices.

Jennifer is an energetic specialist and devotee who has given a very long time to learning new cosmetics strategies, investigating the study of good skin, and incorporating proficient ideas. Her dedication to her own health extends beyond her interest in skin care.

Table of content:

INTRODUCTION... 7
- Introduction to the book and it purpose:................ 7

❖ Purpose for the Book:...................................... 8

● Overview of the importance of skincare and beauty routines:...9

Chapter 1: The Fundamentals of Skin Health........14

● Understanding the science of healthy skin and skincare:... 18

● Identifying factors affecting skin health:...............24

● Healthy beauty habit:...36

Chapter 2: Crafting Your Beauty...............................
Routine.. 49

● Creating a personalized beauty routine:..............67

● Morning and evening routine:.............................. 72

● The role of consistency in skincare:.................... 90

Chapter 3: Embracing Different Skin Types............97

● Identify and understanding various skin types.....98

● Tailoring your skincare routine to your skin type 111

Chapter 4: Common facial Skin Problems............ 149

● Type of acid in Skincare and their benefit:.........150

● Different ingredients in skincare and their benefit...170

● Preventive measures for longterm skin health.. 201

Chapter 5: Mastering Makeup Techniques........... 208

● The correct order of makeup............................. 208

Chapter 6: Staying Ahead of Beauty Trends....... 235

● Tips on staying ahead of beauty trends............235

● Tips to stay healthy conscious while staying on tip of trends..237

Chapter 7: Expert Beauty Advice.........................239

● Insights from skincare and beauty experts........241

Chapter 8: Beauty Secrets Unveiled....................251

● Expert tips for ageless beauty.......................... 253

● Inside beauty hacks...255

● Secret to a healthy lifestyle and nutrition for beauty 257

Chapter 9: Beauty Hacks for Busy Lives.............. 264

● Time saving tricks for a busy lifestyle............... 269

● Maintaining beauty on the go..........................280

Chapter 10:The Cosmetic industry......................284

● Exploring the world of beauty product.............. 285

● Identifying reputable brands and product..........288

● Making informed choice when shopping for cosmetics...294

Chapter 11:A Beauty Journey to Feel your best... 299

● Reflecting your outer beauty............................305

Conclusion: Your path to timeless beauty............311

● Final Thoughts and Encouragement:................ 312

<u>INTRODUCTION</u>

- ## Introduction to the book and it purpose:

Good tidings and welcome to the "New cosmetic beauty and Skincare guide," our manual for magnificence and skincare. This isn't your typical excellence book — rather, a novel one will confer information on themes connecting with magnificence, skincare, and beauty care products as well as unveil tips, stunts, and semi-secret yet intriguing data. In addition, you will receive beauty advice, learn how to create a skincare routine, and apply the most recent cosmetic trends.

❖ Purpose for the Book:

In the event that you've at any point felt like you're not capitalizing on your skin, or that you're investing the effort however not getting results, this book is here to help. It fills in as a twofold asset: in the first place, it offers you the opportunity to gain the best magnificence mysteries from the writing, those in the background tips that truly have an effect, and second, it fills in as an aide for making a skincare routine that works for your skin type as well as stays aware of the quickly impacting universe of excellence patterns.

- **Overview of the importance of skincare and beauty routines:**

Hello! We ought to discuss skincare and beauty routines, which are topics we all enjoy but don't always have time for. It's not just about looking amazing; it's also about feeling fantastic and taking a minute each day to appreciate oneself.

1. Self-Care:A well-done beauty regimen is an act of self-care rather than just vanity. Making time for skincare, haircare, and other grooming practices helps us prioritize self-care in the midst of our busy schedules.

Taking care of our bodies and minds can result in lower stress levels, better mental health, and an all-around increase in self-love.

2.personal expression:

Our beauty routines enable us to use the power of personal style to show our uniqueness and inventiveness. By selecting materials, hues, and styling methods that reflect our tastes, we may show off our individuality and character to the outside world. A beauty regimen allows you to express yourself creatively, whether it's through a signature makeup look, an artfully groomed hairstyle, or just nourished skin.

3. Boosting Self-Confidence:

Taking care of our physical appearance directly affects our perceptions of ourselves and other people. Our self-confidence soars when we feel good about how we look, which has a favorable effect on both our personal and professional life. Maintaining a beauty regimen enables us to present our best selves and emanate confidence from the inside out.

4. Long-Term Advantages:

Maintaining a beauty routine consistently can have amazing long-term effects. For example, regular skincare preserves a young glow, delays the signs of aging, and supports healthy skin. Following a haircare regimen keeps our hair healthy by avoiding damage and encouraging growth. Investing in our future selves by following a beauty routine enhances our inherent qualities and yields enduring advantages.

5. Conscious Self-Evaluation:

Putting a beauty routine into practice is a chance for deliberate introspection and appreciation of oneself. We give ourselves times to be still and mindful of ourselves as we wash, moisturize, or put on makeup. These times can serve as a spark for reflection, helping us to value our physical attributes, pinpoint areas in which we would like to grow, and develop an appreciation for who we are.

Beauty regimens are vital to our general health and well-being; they are not only about looking nice. Putting time and effort into a regular beauty regimen as a means of self-care increases self-esteem, fosters individuality, and increases confidence. Therefore, embrace the power of beauty routines and allow them to bring out your inner glow so that you can shine in all facets of your life. Recall that taking care of oneself is always worthwhile and that your journey toward self-care is what makes you beautiful!

Chapter 1: The Fundamentals of Skin Health.

The basics of skin wellbeing include a mix of good skincare rehearses, a sound way of life, and security against natural elements. Here are a few key basics:

Hydration: Water is your skin's dearest companion. Skin is practically 65% water. Remaining hydrated appears to be legit.

Work out: Exercise jump starts the system. Skin gleaming post-exercise? That is the consequence of an expanded blood stream carrying oxygen to cells. Exercise can likewise lessen tension, which assists with dermatitis, psoriasis and skin break out.

Unwinding: Unwinding quiets everything,Mind, body - and skin. Stress can cause irritation.

Sound eating regimen: Solid eating routine makes sound skin,Taking in the right supplements for your skin. Whole grains, foods grown from the ground support the skin's capability. There's likewise proof that a high-fiber diet works on the standpoint for skin disease patients.

Rest: Rest assists in skin with fixing. Rest is fundamental for fixing cells. That goes for skin as well.

Getting a yearly skin check: Early discovery can fix most types of skin disease - a full-body proficient assessment will reassure you.

Skin protection: What happens outside is essentially as significant as inside. A brilliant skincare system secures and protects the skin, and

Clean up with tepid water: Saturate, as this renews the greasy external layer (lipid obstruction, in the event that we're getting specialized), keeping skin solid. Saturate two times per day

Utilize an enemy of ager, for example, retinoid or L-ascorbic acid serum - particularly significant once you hit your thirties, and then some begin with the least suggested measurement for items with solid dynamic fixings like retinol, and step by step increment so your skin can develop resistance.

Use sunblock with SPF50+ to safeguard against UV beams, which cause untimely maturing and can cause skin malignant growthShed, to eliminate dead skin,and keep your skin solid and sparkling.

Note that few out of every odd kind of shedding might work for each skin type, it's critical to consider your skin type prior to picking a peeling technique and forever be delicate on your skin.

These are the underpinnings of strong skincare. But at the same time it merits remembering the accompanying:

Over washing: It can strip away the defensive greasy external layer of the skin.

Try not to utilize cleanser and hot water .Once more, since they can strip away the external layer.

Grating exfoliants can harm the external layer.Try not to utilize various items at the same time.

- **Understanding the science of healthy skin and skincare:**

The skin isn't just an impression of our general wellbeing yet additionally a material of our magnificence. Understanding the science behind skincare is fundamental for keeping up with sound, brilliant skin. In this article, we will investigate the essentials of skincare and dive into the logical rules that guide our quest for sound skin.

The Skin Hindrance: Your Most memorable Line of Guard

The furthest layer of our skin, known as the epidermis, goes about as an obstruction that safeguards us from hurtful natural elements, including UV radiation, toxins, and organisms. This obstruction is made out of particular skin cells called keratinocytes, which produce an intense protein called keratin. Solid skin depends on a reasonable creation of these cells, and interruptions can prompt different skin conditions.

One critical part of the skin boundary is lipids, including ceramides, cholesterol, and free unsaturated fats. These lipids structure the mortar between the block like keratinocytes, making a water-safe obstruction that forestalls lack of hydration and the passage of microorganisms. Skincare items that contain fixings like ceramides can help backing and fix this indispensable obstruction, keeping your skin hydrated and safeguarded.

The Job of pH in Skincare

The pH level of your skin is a central component that impacts its wellbeing. The skin's pH preferably drifts around 4.5 to 5.5, making it somewhat acidic. This corrosiveness is fundamental since it keeps up with the skin hindrance and represses the development of unsafe microorganisms. Utilizing unforgiving cleaning agents or basic skincare items can disturb this sensitive equilibrium, prompting skin dryness and bothering.

Understanding your skin's pH and picking skincare items that regard this regular sharpness is urgent. It guarantees that your skin stays in its ideal condition and can really safeguard against outside stressors. Continuously check the pH levels of your chemicals and toners to guarantee they are viable with your skin's necessities.

The Force of Cancer prevention agents.
One of the main dangers to your skin's wellbeing is oxidative pressure, which results from an unevenness between free revolutionaries and cell reinforcements in your body. Free revolutionaries are unsteady atoms that can harm skin cells, prompting untimely maturing and different skin issues. Cell reinforcements, then again, assist with killing these unsafe particles and safeguard your skin.

Nutrients C and E are notable cancer prevention agents that assume an imperative part in skincare. L-ascorbic acid lights up the skin and animates collagen creation, decreasing the presence of almost negligible differences. Vitamin E, a fat-solvent cell reinforcement, attempts to shield the skin from UV harm and natural contaminations. Remembering items rich for cell reinforcements in your skincare routine can assist with combatting the impacts of oxidative pressure and keep your skin looking energetic.

The Advantages of Retinoids

Retinoids are subordinates of vitamin An and are viewed as one of the highest quality levels in skincare.Using brutal cleaning agents or soluble skincare items can upset this sensitive equilibrium, prompting skin dryness and disturbance.

Understanding your skin's pH and picking skincare items that regard this normal causticity is urgent. It guarantees that your skin stays in its ideal condition and can actually safeguard against outer stressors. Continuously check the pH levels of your cleaning agents and toners to guarantee they are viable with your skin's requirements.

The Significance of Hydration

Skin hydration is a foundation of solid skin. At the point when your skin is enough saturated, it stays stout, flexible, and better prepared to avoid harm from ecological stressors. Got dried out skin, then again, can prompt barely recognizable differences, a dull coloring, and an expanded powerlessness to bothering. To keep up with skin hydration, it's vital to utilize a lotion reasonable for your skin type. For those with dry skin, heavier, oil-based creams are gainful, while people with slick skin ought to settle on lightweight, non-comedogenic choices. Moreover, drinking a satisfactory measure of water is fundamental to guarantee your skin stays all around hydrated from the inside.

• Identifying factors affecting skin health:

1.Age

Understanding the effects that maturing has on your skin will help you loads. With time, your skin:

Becomes more slender, making veins Gives more slow indications of recovery and reestablishment noticeable and pores bigger

Holds less water, hence evaporating and drying out without any problem

Begins wrinkling and listing

Dials back on collagen creation, hence missing out on versatility

The circumstance could appear to be really sad, and tragically, we have no cheerful astonishments to toss your direction. Be that as it may, following a reliably effective skincare routine will help maturing. We guarantee. Tip: Recall that skincare in your 20's will to a great extent reflect in later phases of your life.

2. Skin Type

skin type is the venturing stone to accomplishing perfect skin. It is additionally conceivable that your skin type changes with moving seasons and conditions. Independent, this is the way skin types influence your skin:

Dry Skin: Successive tingling and flakiness, unpleasantness, inclination to break particularly around winters, prior indications of maturing and wrinkling.

Oily Skin: Skin break out inclined, obviously apparent and frequently developed pores, issues of hyper pigmentation.

Combination Skin: Flakiness in winter environments, obstructed pores and skin inflammation, and a ton of disarray.

Normal Skin: By and large even; yet frequently gets drier with maturing.

Know that regardless of your skin type, there's a correct method for really focusing on it.

3. Identity

This one's fairly less spoken about, yet really intriguing. Your ethnic starting points impact the construction and presence of your skin and how your skin responds to the sun, causing various degrees of sun harm.

It has been shown that hazier skin (consider individuals Hispanic, African starting points) contains more melanin - the color that gives skin its regular complexion. This goes about as both a gift and a revile - on one hand, the skin is better shielded from UV beams, subsequently deferring indications of maturing. On the other, pigmentation issues become more significant.

On the other hand, age spots are more apparent on Caucasian and Southwest Asian skins than on hazier skin types. Besides, because of their craving for tanning, dangers to skin disease are higher.

4. Normal Complexion

An outing to the ocean side could make you can't help thinking about why certain individuals get burns from the sun, and some get suntans. Your normal complexion is one of the key factors that influence your skin. Yet again we should discuss melanin.

In more obscure complexions, a higher melanin content safeguards the skin from sun harm and makes it tan. To this end more obscure cleaned individuals generally turn hazier or tan on going through hours in the sun.

In lighter complexions, a lower melanin content leads one to become red or consume when they go out in the sun.

Regardless of your complexion, we'd encourage you to never relinquish your cherished sunscreen bottle. In some cases, tenacious is perfect!

5. Stress

Today, we're very mindful of the irrefutable connection between the psychological and the physical. At the point when stress assumes control over you, your body will undoubtedly answer. Sadly, the skin is no exemption. Stress prompts hormonal changes, which thus cause skin inflammation breakouts. Besides, things are in many cases exacerbated by unreasonable sweat, overconsumption of dehydrators like espresso and liquor, deficient rest, and a dismissed skincare schedule.

6. Rest Cycle

Skincare specialists have consistently focused on the significance of rest. We might want to repeat that by saying - magnificence rest is genuine. While you're dozing ceaselessly in brilliance, your skin is on to some serious work. Development chemicals help fix and recharge harmed skin cells, and hydration and collagen levels are reestablished. Moreover, absence of rest additionally speeds up skin illnesses like dermatitis and psoriasis. Thus, the following time somebody considers you a resting delight, explain to them why you love your rest.

7. Water Utilization

This enchanted mixture called water is in a real sense one of the most compelling things that influence your skin. Overall, the human body is 60% water. Enormous amounts of water are lost from the body consistently. On the off chance that the sufficient substitution doesn't happen, difficult issues come to the front. Drinking sufficient water (no less than 8 glasses every day) will dispense with your requirement for various skincare items. Less kinks, more clear coloring, quicker mending, more modest pores, more tight skin, diminished puffiness, less skin inflammation, and the rundown goes on.

8. Your Current circumstance

Where do you burn through a large portion of your day? Is it bound to cooled spaces, or outside - in the sun? Very few might know this, yet the natural factors that influence skin are really destructive.

Outside: Extended periods of UV openness can cause burns from the sun, rashes, redness, and higher dangers of skin malignant growth. Additionally, note that the sun is never not there. SPF sunscreens are your dearest companion even on cloudy days.

Inside: A forced air system works by drawing out heat from the air inside the room, and tossing it outside. Sadly, it isn't adequately prepared to separate between dampness in the air and that on your skin. This makes the skin dry, tight, and got dried out.

9. Way of life Variables

All of us are various people, as are our ways of life. This is the way specific sorts of ways of life manifest themselves in our skins' wellbeing.

Continuous Voyaging: Travel is a ton about managing changes - be it your timetable, the air, the climate, or your skincare schedule. To this end breakouts while voyaging are normal.

Diet: You truly are what you eat. Eating food varieties wealthy in supplements and cancer prevention agents will show on your skin. Question us? Attempt it!

Work Out: Working it out helps discharge poisons and pollutions from the body. This is positively perfect for the skin and accomplishes clear appearances. Nonetheless, it is important to purge the skin post working out.

Liquor: as well as being a pleasant expansion to gatherings and parties, liquor is likewise a known dehydrator. Inordinate utilization of alcohol peels the skin off of the dampness that it needs.

Smoking: Every individual who smokes routinely knows about its damages. For clear reasons, smoking likewise makes extensive harm the skin. It has been for quite some time related with untimely maturing, wrinkling, drying out, and in additional extreme cases, skin disease.

10. Cosmetics

For some's purposes, cosmetics use is just incidental. Nonetheless, many use it consistently. Exorbitant utilization of cosmetics speeds up issues of skin break out, untimely maturing, sensitivities, and discolouration. Independent of whether you use cosmetics sporadically, frequently, or consistently, ensure you avoid potential risk. Keep brushes clean, stay away from destructive fixings, realize your skin type, and become friends with facial cleaning agents.

Your skin is made to tolerate a ton of stressors. This can absolutely make it hard to anticipate what precisely your skin needs. Subsequently starts a section of vast detailed trials.

To let you free from all the mystery, we at Yours have concocted coordinating your skin needs with a customized skincare schedule. Our items are supported by genuine science and are 100 percent brutality free. Moreover, they represent all of the previously mentioned natural, ecological, and way of life factors.

- **Healthy beauty habit:**

This are some solid excellence propensity to rehearse for your skin upgrade.

1.Not Contacting Your Face:

Contacting your face continually can spread infections, microorganisms and allergens; all of which can cause breakouts or aggravate skin.

2.Hydrate from The inside:

Drinking a lot of water isn't just significant for your general wellbeing yet in addition for the soundness of your skin. Aim to drink no less than 8 glasses of water a day and increment your admission on the off chance that you are practicing or in a hot place.

3.Rest:

 helps in keeping up with the wellbeing and presence of your skin. Absence of rest can prompt bluntness, puffiness, and dark circles under the eyes.

4. Scrub, Tone, and Saturate:

A reliable skincare routine is fundamental for keeping up with sound skin. Begin by purifying your face two times every day to eliminate soil, oil, and pollutions that can obstruct your pores. Pick a chemical that is reasonable for your skin type, whether it's sleek, dry, or mix. Subsequent to purging, circle back to a toner to adjust the pH of your skin and eliminate even the slightest hints of soil. At last, saturate your skin to keep it hydrated and graceful. Search for a cream that is reasonable for your skin type and contains fixings that support and safeguard your skin.

4. Safeguard with Sunscreen:

Sun insurance is pivotal for keeping up with the wellbeing and energy of your skin. The destructive UV beams from the sun can cause untimely maturing, kinks, and sunspots. Apply a wide range sunscreen with a SPF of something like 30 consistently, even on overcast days. Remember to reapply sunscreen like clockwork, particularly on the off chance that you are investing energy outside. Moreover, wearing defensive attire, like caps and shades, can additionally protect your skin from the sun's destructive beams.

5. Eat a Fair Eating regimen:

Eating a reasonable eating regimen wealthy in organic products, vegetables, lean proteins, and sound fats furnishes your skin with the supplements it necessities to remain solid and brilliant. Cancer prevention agent rich food sources, like berries, tomatoes, and mixed greens, assist with battling free extremists and shield your skin from harm. Stay away from handled food varieties, sweet tidbits, and exorbitant liquor utilization, as these can add to irritation and breakouts.

6. Workout Consistently:

Customary activity helps your general wellbeing as well as your skin. At the point when you work out, your pulse increments, advancing better blood dissemination all through your body, including your skin. This expanded blood stream conveys oxygen and supplements to your skin cells, giving you a sound shine. Practice likewise assists with diminishing pressure, which can emphatically affect your skin. Hold back nothing 30 minutes of moderated force work out, like lively strolling or swimming, most days of the week.

7. Try not to Smoke and Restrict Liquor Utilization:

Smoking stances serious wellbeing gambles as well as negatively affects your skin. Smoking strait the veins in your skin, lessening blood stream and oxygen supply. This can prompt a dull tone, wrinkles, and an expanded gamble of skin malignant growth. Essentially, inordinate liquor utilization can get dried out your skin and cause irritation.

8. Practice Great Cleanliness:

Keeping up with great cleanliness propensities is fundamental for solid skin. Continuously eliminate your cosmetics prior to hitting the hay to permit your skin to inhale and forestall stopped up pores. Utilize delicate, non disturbing chemicals and keep away from unforgiving cleaning, which can harm your skin. Change your pillowcases consistently to keep away from the development of soil and microscopic organisms. Furthermore, try not to contact your face over the course of the day to forestall the exchange of microbes and soil from your hands onto your skin.

9. Look for Proficient Exhortation:

While these day to day propensities can incredibly work on the wellbeing and presence of your skin, it's memorable essential that everybody's skin is one of a kind. In the event that you have explicit skin concerns or conditions, it's ideal to look for proficient guidance from a dermatologist or skin health management trained professional.

10. Take a stab at utilizing a serum:

Serums are an incredible method for giving your skin an additional lift. They contain concentrated fixings that can help hydrate, light up, and smooth your skin.

All in all, why not have a go at utilizing a serum consistently and perceive how your skin answers? You may simply be shocked at the outcomes.

11.Throw away obsolete cosmetics as well as skincare items:

It's not only a decent stunner propensity to toss out obsolete items - it's really a significant security safeguard. On the off chance that you don't have the foggiest idea about the lapse date of an item, search for the open container image on the bundling. That will let you know how long it's protected to utilize the item before you ought to dispose of it.

All things considered, lapsed cosmetics and skincare items can contain microorganisms that can prompt skin diseases or different issues. It's simply not worth the gamble - thus, best to be as cautious as possible!

12.Regularly clean your cosmetics and skincare devices:

Cosmetics brushes, wipes, tweezers, and that multitude of different instruments we use for our excellence schedules are inclined to gathering microbes. Therefore it's so essential to clean them consistently and appropriately. If not, you could be bringing microorganisms into your skin each time you use them.

13.Be predictable with your skincare schedule:

An incredible skincare routine is just pretty much as viable as your consistency. In the event that you're just utilizing your items each now and, it'll be a lot harder to see the outcomes you need - and your skin will not be as sound by the same token.

Thus, make a point to adhere to your daily practice! Like that, you can receive its full rewards, and really see the outcomes you're later.

14. Know which skincare fixings to search for:

With regards to skincare, not all fixings are made equivalent. Rather than simply going after any old item off the rack, instruct yourself on which fixings are awesome for your skin type - and pay special attention to them

15. Try not to pop your zits:

Let's be real, I'm awful for this - and consistently have been. In any case, it's really an extremely persistent vice to get into!

Popping your zits can prompt skin issues, for example, scarring and contamination. Additionally, it can harm the fragile skin around and underneath the pimple. In this way, rather than popping or picking at your skin break out, settle on a delicate spot treatment all things considered Or, even better, go see a dermatologist.

16.Always play out a fix test first with any new items:

It doesn't make any difference how much your companion goes on and on about a specific item; you ought to continuously make certain to play out a fix test first. It's the most ideal way to ensure that the item is reasonable for your skin type, and won't bring about any responses or disturbance.

You should simply apply a limited quantity of the item to your skin and sit tight for 24-48 hours. In the event that there's no response, utilizing on your face ought to be protected. Simply remember to apply a cream a short time later!

17. Indulge yourself with a facial covering:

We as a whole realize that a facial covering can be an incredible method for giving your skin an additional lift. They're likewise really unwinding, which generally assists with lessening pressure and advance sound skin.

In the event that you need greatest outcomes, settle on an earth veil! They work best to clean your skin, draw out pollutions, and even control abundance oil. Moreover, you can likewise find facial coverings with other stalwart fixings, as well - like L-ascorbic acid or hyaluronic corrosive.

18. Take a skincare course so you can all the more likely grasp your skin:
Understanding your skin is quite possibly of the most ideal option for it. Taking a skincare course will assist you with more deeply studying your skin type, what fixings are best for you, and how to take legitimate consideration of it - in a tomfoolery and intelligent way.

Chapter 2: Crafting Your Beauty Routine

Do you feel tired when people talk about their skincare routine? How many times have you watched several videos and when you hear them mention some expensive products, you give up? Or you end up using and it does not work for you.Hold on! The steps to crafting a skincare routine that is suited just for you are not only simple but worthwhile.

Are you ready? I'm sure you are so keep reading.

How to Create a Skincare Schedule That Works for You

1 Recognizing the Particular Requirements of Your Skin
a How to Determine Your Skin Type:
b Skin ailments:
Evaluating Your Skin Objectives:
2 Creating a Customized Skincare Program
3. Giving Less Ingredients and No Fragrance Priority
Four Possible Triggers to Watch Out for
5. The Effectiveness of Simplified Formulations

Six Synopsis

The secret to having clear, smooth skin is creating a skincare regimen that suits your needs and tastes and works well. It's easy to feel overwhelmed by the sheer number of products available, but developing a customized skincare routine can be simple and satisfying.

This post will explain how to create a skincare routine that uses only natural chemicals and enhances your skin's inherent radiance.

1 Grasping Your Skin's Extraordinary Requirements

Prior to jumping into the points of interest of your skincare schedule, understanding your skin's remarkable characteristics is fundamental. This information frames the establishment whereupon you'll assemble a viable daily schedule. Begin by recognizing your skin type:

A. Recognizing Your Skin Type:

Skin type alludes to how much sebum created by your sebaceous organs.

Oily: Assuming that your skin will in general be sparkly and inclined to breakouts.

Dry: On the off chance that your skin feels tight, flaky, and needs dampness.

Combination: In the event that you have a blend of oily and dry regions.

Normal: Assuming that your skin feels adjusted and agreeable.

B. Skin conditions:

In fact talking, any skin type is defenseless to these skin conditions.

Delicate: Assuming that your skin responds to items with redness, tingling, or disturbance.

Got dried out: Assuming that your skin feels dry, tight, and needs dampness yet gives indications of slickness and clog, it very well might be dried out. This condition concerns an absence of water, not oil, and can influence any skin type.

Skin inflammation inclined: Skin break out inclined skin alludes to a skin type that is especially helpless to creating skin inflammation, a typical skin condition portrayed by the presence of pimples, zits, whiteheads, and once in a while significantly more significant, excruciating knobs. As a rule, skin break out inclined skin is related with slick and delicate skin.

C. Evaluating Your Skin Objectives:

While choosing skincare items, taking into account your particular goals is fundamental. Is it true that you are focusing on skin inflammation, scarce differences, or just hoping to keep a solid coloring? Knowing your skincare objectives will direct you in picking the most fitting items and elements for your everyday practice.

2 Making Your Customized Skincare Schedule
Purifying - A Delicate Beginning:

Start with a delicate cleaning agent fit to your skin type. Purifying eliminates soil, cosmetics, and contaminations, making way for successful skincare. My most loved is this hydrating cleaning agent from Cerave. It's reasonable for all skin types, delicate, and aroma free.

Twofold purging around evening time:

Twofold purging, a foundation of powerful skincare, includes a two step purifying cycle that guarantees your skin is completely spotless and prepared to ingest the advantages of resulting skincare items. The strategy began in Korean skincare schedules and has acquired prevalence overall for its capacity to profoundly scrub and revive the skin.

The initial step regularly includes utilizing an oil based cleaning agent to eliminate cosmetics, sunscreen, and abundance oil. This underlying wash separates debasements that can amass on your skin's surface over the course of the day.

The subsequent step utilizes a water based cleaning agent to eliminate the excess buildup and give a more profound scrub. By taking part in twofold purifying, you're eliminating soil and poisons and making way for your skincare items to enter all the more actually, upgrading their general effect.

This strategy is essential in metropolitan conditions, for sunscreen evacuation, or subsequent to wearing cosmetics, as it keeps up with the wellbeing and brilliance of your skin by forestalling blockage and permitting it to openly relax.

Integrating twofold purifying into your skincare routine can raise your taking care of oneself custom, leaving your skin revived, renewed, and prepared to retain the decency of your picked skincare.

Shedding - Banishing Dead Skin Cells:

Peeling your skin no less than once a month is my proposal to dispose of dead skin cells. While week by week peeling is recommended, numerous skincare items as of now have shedding properties. Furthermore, a washcloth can physically peel your skin, so you should not do it as frequently as you naturally suspect.

A decent choice is compound exfoliants with glycolic or salicylic corrosive. In the event that you have delicate skin, a PHA exfoliant might be the best approach since they are regularly not as bothering. At the present time, I favor utilizing spicules to physically peel my skin.

Marine wipes called spicules have hostile to bacterial and calming properties and are additionally insignificantly rough. These spicules can enter profound into the skin and invigorate collagen creation. This interaction is frequently contrasted with miniature needling.

Hydration - Extinguishing Your Skin's Thirst:

Hydration is crucial, no matter what your skin type. A hydrating serum or quintessence containing hyaluronic acid can assist your skin with holding dampness. My most loved hyaluronic acid serum is this one.

Treatment - Focusing on Unambiguous Worries:

Assuming that you have concerns like skin inflammation, maturing, or hyperpigmentation, consolidate designated medicines.

Moisturizing - Fixing in Goodness:

Secure in hydration with a cream suitable for your skin type — even slick skin benefits from lightweight, sans oil lotions.

Sun Assurance - Safeguarding Your Skin:

Never skip sunscreen, even on shady days. Decide on a wide range sunscreen with essentially SPF 50 to safeguard against destructive UV beams. I favor Korean sunscreens since they are more thorough than American ones.

Understand this: My day to day sunscreen schedule.

3 Focusing on Insignificant Fixings and Zero Aroma
Fixing Awareness:

Picking items with insignificant fixings decreases the gamble of possible aggravations. Throughout recent years, we've heard numerous popular expressions like "clean fixings" and "clean young lady tasteful." While I concur with parts of that way of thinking, a few issues emerge with items considered as "clean."

The "spotless" development has altogether affected our impression of additives. Because of steady air, water, and human contact openness, healthy skin items expect additives to forestall microbes development.

Besides, skincare items require a few additives to keep them from having a considerably more limited timeframe of realistic usability than they presently do. To assist with everything going on, many organizations supplant customary additives with fixings like methylisothiazolinone, known to be an aggravation.

Besides, some "perfect fixing" items get that name since they use plant botanicals and natural ointments, which likewise disturb an enormous populace.

Thus, fixing awareness includes cautiously looking at the parts of your skin health management items and guaranteeing they line up with your skin's requirements. Choosing items with negligible, very much picked fixings lessens the gamble of likely disturbances and advances a better, more brilliant tone.

4 Possible Aggravations to Search For:
While the skincare world offers a variety of botanicals and mixtures, not all fixings are all around very much endured. Natural balms, frequently utilized for their fragrant characteristics, can be possible aggravations for some people, causing redness, tingling, or hypersensitive responses.

Plants inferred botanicals, while normal, can likewise hold onto allergenic mixtures that lead to responsive qualities. It's vital for watch for these fixings, particularly assuming that you have delicate or effectively receptive skin.

Medicinal balms: Rejuvenating ointments like citrus, lavender, and peppermint might sharpen a few people. While they can offer advantages in certain examples, they can likewise set off unfriendly responses in others. Settle on scent free items to keep away from possible aggravations.

Plant Botanicals: Despite the fact that plant based fixings are mending, practicing caution is fundamental. Plant concentrates can set off sensitivities or aggravations in people with delicate skin.

All the more critically, these unfavorable responses are bound to slip through the cracks as the rashes would happen haphazardly. It is fitting to fix test new items that contain plants inferred fixings before completely integrating them into your skincare schedule.

5 The Force of Moderate Definitions:
Looking for items with less fixings can fundamentally decrease the probability of skin responses. Moderate details frequently center around center parts that address explicit skincare worries without presenting superfluous intricacies.

Search for items that focus on dynamic fixings valuable to your skin types, for example, hyaluronic corrosive for hydration, niacinamide for lighting up, and ceramides for hindrance support.

Aroma Free Advantages:

Aroma can cause awareness and aggravation, in any event, for those without delicate skin. Choosing scent free items limits the gamble of antagonistic responses.

Fix Testing:

Continuously play out a fix test on a little skin region while acquainting new items with guarantee similarity and forestall likely unfavorably susceptible responses.

Summary:

Creating a skincare routine custom made to your skin's extraordinary requirements is a strong method for upgrading your normal magnificence and lift your certainty. Keep in mind, straightforwardness is critical - center around fundamental stages and negligible elements for ideal outcomes.

By integrating items that line up with your skin type, objectives, and inclinations, you're in route to supporting your skin and encountering the sparkle from the inside. Host your skincare process with a customized schedule that causes you to feel brilliant and certain day to day.

- **Creating a personalized beauty routine:**

Whether you want to smooth wrinkles, fade brown spots, or shrink your pores, what and how you use it depends on your individual skin type and skincare needs.

Read on to find out how to build your own personalized skincare routine and get the best skin of your life.

Your personalized skincare routine starts with a basic regimen plus products formulated for your specific skin type (oily, dry, combination, etc.). Start with

1.cleanser, then follow it with
2.exfoliant, and finish with
3.moisturizer with SPF for day and moisturizer without SPF for night.

Now that you've established a foundation, you can further personalize your routine by adding in one or more of the following skincare champions:

Toners

Toners are often the unsung heroes of a skincare routine. The right toner can breathe new life into a lackluster complexion. Use a toner after cleansing as the second step in your skincare routine. Toners with antioxidants and skin repairing ingredients (hyaluronic acid, glycerin, ceramides, and fatty acids) will not only remove the last traces of makeup but also will provide benefits targeted to your specific skin concerns. The right toner will leave your skin smoother, soothe redness, and even help improve the appearance of enlarged pores. Even better, that the right toner contains more of these ingredients than many serums or moisturizers

Antioxidant serums

The best antioxidant serums not only contain high concentrations of potent antioxidants (think vitamin C, resveratrol, green tea extract and more), but they are also loaded with cell communicating ingredients (think niacinamide and retinol). When you begin using a serum you'll see improvements right away as their antioxidant-rich formulas soothe redness and brighten skin. Over the long term you'll see signs of aging fade and skin will look and feel healthier and firmer, too! Use your serum after your exfoliant.

Masks

A mask or other facial treatment is ideal for addressing a special need or occasional concern such as adding extra hydration, absorbing excess oil, or calming redness.

Boosters

Sometimes your skin needs a bit of extra TLC. That's where anti aging boosters come in. Each booster targets a specific skin care concern and can easily be added to your skincare routine. Combine a few drops with your serum or moisturizer.

By adding the above products, your routine will look something like this:

* ❖ Cleanser

* ❖ Toner

* ❖ Exfoliant (AHA or BHA)

* ❖ Booster

* ❖ Antioxidant serum and/or targeted treatment

* ❖ Day Moisturizer with SPF / Night Moisturiser (without SPF)

- **Morning and evening routine:**

Your skin care routine is an important part of every day. If you use multiple products morning and evening, the order you use them matters.

What Order Should I Follow for My Skin Care Routine?

What should I use in the morning?

Morning skin care routines are all about prevention and protection. Your face is going to be exposed to the outside environment, so necessary steps include moisturizer and sunscreen.

• Basic morning routine

Cleanser: Use it to remove grime and residue that's built up overnight.

Moisturizer: This hydrates the skin and can come in the form of creams, gels, or balms.

Sunscreen: It's essential for protecting the skin against the damaging effects of the sun.

Was this helpful?

Step 1: Oil based cleanser:

It is intended to dissolve oils produced by your skin.

Step 2: Water based cleanser:

These cleansers primarily contain surfactants, which are ingredients that allow water to rinse away dirt and sweat. They can also remove the oils collected by an oil based cleanser. Skip this step if You don't want to double cleanse or if your oil based cleanser contains surfactants that sufficiently remove dirt and debris.

Look for a cleanser with a neutral or low pH,a Mild water based cleansers may help prevent breakouts in those with acne prone or oily skin.

Step 3: Toner or astringent
Toners are designed to replenish skin through hydration and remove dead cells and dirt left behind after cleansing. An astringent is an alcohol based product used to remove excess

oil. Avoid toners high in alcohol as they can irritate your skin.

Step 4: Antioxidant serum
Serums contain a high concentration of certain ingredients. An antioxidant-based serum will protect skin against damage caused by unstable molecules known as free radicals. Vitamins C and E are common antioxidants used to improve texture and firmness. Others to look out for include green tea, resveratrol, and caffeine,use serum that will protect you against ultraviolet A (UVA) and ultraviolet B (UVB) rays and lessen signs of aging. Test a new product in a small area to see how it works on your skin and with the other products in your routine.

Some serums, such as those that contain acids, may cause irritation when combined with other acid containing skin care products.

Step 5: Spot treatment

If you have a blemish with a head, first look for an anti inflammatory product to remove it, then turn to a spot drying treatment to clear up the rest. Anything under the skin is classified as a cyst and will require a product that targets the infection on the inside.

Skip this step if You have no spots or want to let nature take its course.

Always introduce a new product slowly and monitor your skin.

Step 6: Eye cream

The skin around your eyes tends to be thinner and more sensitive. It's also prone to signs of aging, including fine lines, puffiness, and darkness. A good eye cream can brighten, smooth, and firm up the area, but it won't completely eliminate issues.

Skip this step if Your moisturizer and serum are suitable for the eye area, contain an effective formula, and are fragrances free.

Step 7: Lighter face oil

The lighter the product, the earlier you should apply it. Easily absorbable oils are lightweight and should therefore come before moisturizer. They're especially useful if your skin's showing signs of dryness, flakiness, or dehydration. More often than not, you'll have to try different oils to see which works best for you.

Be sure to Let your oil sink in fully before applying sunscreen. Some face oils may dissolve your sunscreen.

The Oils may cause breakouts in people with oily skin.

Step 8: Moisturizer

A moisturizer will soothe and soften skin. If you have a dry skin type, opt for a cream or balm. Thicker creams work best on normal or combination skin, and fluids and gels are recommended for oilier types. Effective ingredients include glycerine, ceramides, antioxidants, and peptides.

Skip this step if Your toner or serum gives you enough moisture. This is especially true for those with oily skin. Be sure to Apply moisturizer with clean hands — especially if you're using it from a jar that you dip your fingers into. If you use dirty hands, you may be adding dirt and even bacteria into your moisturizer.

Step 9: Heavier face oil

Oils that take some time to absorb or simply feel thick fall into the heavy category. Best suited for dry skin types, these should be applied after moisturizer to seal in all the goodness. Skip this step if You don't want to run the risk of clogging your pores. Again, trial and error is key here.

Be sure to Fully cleanse your face at the end of the day, as heavier face oils can contribute to clogging pores.

Step 10: Sunscreen

Sunscreen is a critical final step in your morning skin care routine. Not only can it lower your risk of skin cancer, but it can also reduce signs of aging by blocking damaging UV light. The American Cancer SocietyTrusted Source recommends choosing a broad spectrum sunblock rated SPF 30 or higher that protects against UVA and UVB light.

Be sure to Reapply sunblock to your face and body every 2 hours while spending time in the sun.

Using sunblock along with taking other precautions like wearing a hat and being in the shade can help lower your risk for skin cancer. Some sunscreens may cause skin reactions, so it is important to test in a small area prior to applying over the body. Other formulas may not be safe for marine life, such as the coral reef, if you will be swimming in ocean water. Be sure to read the label to determine the best product for your needs.

Step 11: Foundation

Foundation or other base makeup If you want to wear makeup, a base layer will give you a smooth, even complexion. Opt for foundation — which comes in a cream, liquid, or powder form — or a lightweight tinted moisturizer or BB cream.

Skip this step if You prefer to go all natural. Be sure to Check your foundation's expiration date. Many last for 6 to 12 months from the date you first open them.

What should I use at night?
Focus on repairing the damage done during the day with thicker products at night. This is also the time to use anything that makes skin sensitive to sunlight, including physical exfoliants and chemical peels.

- **Night routine**

Cosmetics remover:It does what it says on the tin, in any event, eliminating the cosmetics buildup you can't see.

Cleanser: This will remove any thing that clog your pores.

Spot treatment:You can really treat breakouts around evening time with calming and drying items.

Night cream or rest cover:A more extravagant lotion helps with skin fix.

Was this useful?

Stage 1: Oil based cosmetics remover.

As well as dissolving the regular oils created by your skin, an oil-based cleaning agent can separate sleek fixings found. Skip this step in the event that You don't wear cosmetics, have slick skin, or would like to utilize a water based item.

Make certain to peruse the guidelines on your oil based cosmetics remover, as some might guide you to follow this step with one more kind of chemical or micellar water to eliminate buildup.

Stage 2: Water based cleanser

Water based cleanser respond with cosmetics and soil on the skin in a manner that permits all that to be flushed away with water.

Stage 3: Exfoliator

Peeling eliminates dead skin cells while clearing pores. Mud veils work to unclog pores, yet can likewise retain overabundance oil. These covers are best applied around evening time to eliminate extra soil and assist the skin with absorbing different items.

Stage 4: Hydrating fog or toner

A hydrating fog or toner denotes the finish of your evening time purging daily schedule.

you ought to pay special attention to humectant fixings — lactic acid, hyaluronic acid,and glycerine — to truly give skin a dampness support.

Make certain to Stay away from abuse of toners with elevated degrees of alcohols, as they might make bothering or harm your skin's barrier. Alcohol based items might cause aggravation in people with delicate skin.

Stage 5: acid treatment

Splashing your face in acid might sound unnerving, yet this skin health management treatment can empower cell turnover. Amateurs might need to attempt glycolic acid. Different choices incorporate like for skin break out - salicylic acid and for dry skin- hyaluronic acid . After some time, you ought to see a more splendid and all the more even coloring. Begin once each week fully intent on utilizing consistently. Do a fix test something like 24 hours before first use. Add a couple of drops of the answer for a cotton cushion and clear across the face. Try to keep away from the eye area. Skip this step assuming that You have especially delicate skin or experience a response to a specific acid. Be sure to Pick an acid treatment that meets your skin's requirements.

Acids might make your skin more delicate to the sun. Make certain to utilize sunblock during the day following use of a acid treatment.

Stage 6: Serums and substances

Serums convey strong fixings straightforwardly to the skin. A pith is essentially a watered-down form. Vitamin E is perfect for dry skin, while cell reinforcements like green tea concentrate can be utilized on dull appearances. In the event that you're inclined to breakouts, attempt retinol or L-ascorbic acid.

Make certain to Pick a serum that conveys helps your skin needs, whether one spotlights on favorable to maturing support, saturating, lighting up, or spot decrease.

Step7: Spot treatment

Mitigating items are for flaws with a head. Follow with a spot drying treatment. Ones that dry noticeably are perfect for evening us. Avoid this step if. You're without spot.

Make certain to Try not to pop pimples, imperfections, and whiteheads yourself. The AAD says that this can cause scarring, present microorganisms, and drive discharge further under the skin. In the event that you don't see improvement in 4 to about a month and a half, think about conversing with a dermatologist.

Stage 8: Hydrating serum

A few items can obstruct pores, yet hydrating serums aren't one of them. With the capacity to sneak up suddenly, they're great for dry skin.

Stage 9: Eye cream

 A more extravagant evening eye cream can assist with further developing appearance related issues, similar to sleepiness and scarcely discernible differences. Search for a high convergence of peptides and cell reinforcements.

Avoid this step if Your lotion or serum can be securely and really utilized under your eyes.

Stage 10: Face oil

An evening time oil is perfect for dry or got dried out skin. The night is the best opportunity to apply thicker oils that might result in an undesirable sparkly complexion. Be sure to clean completely the next morning to eliminate buildup from heavier items.

A heavier oil may not be the best fit for those with sleek skin or skin break out. Everybody's skin is unique, so track down an item that works for you.

Stage 11: Night cream or rest veil

A Night creams are an absolutely discretionary last step, however they can be beneficial. While day creams are intended to safeguard the skin, these rich lotions assist cell with fixing. Rest covers, then again, seal in the entirety of your different items and contain hydrating fixings sufficiently gentle to be kept on for the time being.

Avoid this step assuming that Your skin as of now looks and feels its ideal. Certain individuals dislike the vibe of laying down with heavier items on. In the event that that is the situation, you can in any case exploit a more lightweight recipe.

- **The role of consistency in skincare:**

The significance of a skincare schedule that is reliable couldn't possibly be more significant - the consistent responsibility prompts groundbreaking outcomes.

With regards to skincare, consistency is vital! It's nothing unexpected, particularly living in a culture that gives us everything quickly, that we need to see those moment results from skincare However focusing on our skin remains something to show restraint toward.

Evaluating recent fads, new brands as well as the typical experimentation of organizing a skincare schedule that works for you, is absolutely ordinary and changes are normal to a great extent, however it's so critical to take note of that lethargy with your skincare routine is one thing that won't ever deliver any outcomes! It's OK to switch things up occasionally, yet adhering to a reliable routine is so key!

We should likewise rapidly discuss having sensible objectives for yourself with regards to your skin and skincare overall. Skin smoothing web-based entertainment channels and face tuning make them think smooth, pore less skin is the standard, yet let me stop you in that general area. IT'S NOT! In all actuality, genuine skin has surface, maturing is totally regular, and everybody is unique! This excursion is particularly your own, so don't allow the unreasonable guidelines to set by society provide you with a ridiculous vision of what this ought to resemble for you. Now is the right time to feel far better in your own skin!

With that being all said, realize that sensible outcomes are conceivable! Skincare is a certain something, alongside sustenance, hydration, and exercise, that will assist you with crawling nearer to that gleaming, stout skin we as a whole longing. In any case, I'll say it once more consistency is Vital! So we should jump into this somewhat more.

It's so essential to take note of that your skin works around evening time to fix itself so you really want to do your part to eliminate your cosmetics and apply your skincare items (as numerous or as not many as that might be) to permit your skin to go about its business while you rest!

Remember that skincare is definitely not an enchanted elixir!! This implies that noticeable outcomes will not simply work out pretty much by accident! Saturating infrequently doesn't consider a skincare schedule, and unfortunately your poor, dry skin won't ever see long haul benefits without responsibility.

Consider IT… Assuming YOU Turned OUT FOR 2 DAYS, Could YOU Get more fit? And A MONTH? Presently WE'RE GETTING Some place!
Consistency with skincare doesn't need to be a gigantic weight! We as a whole carry on with occupied lives and frequently it's so natural to skirt these significant pieces of our day, yet truly consistency just means a couple of moments in the first part of the day and the night. Everything necessary for perfect skin is a couple of brief minutes!

When you start continually adhering to a skincare schedule, you will not have the option to live without it! You'll see that out of nowhere, that bothersome, overwhelming routine will turn into a non debatable and you'll really anticipate those couple of moments of "personal time" every morning and night. So transforming this into a propensity is so significant!

best facial lotion for skin health management At last, here's a couple of straightforward tips to assist you with remaining reliable

Keep an update by your toothbrush

Set an update on your telephone

Make a taking care of oneself custom out of it with the goal that it seems more like a treat than a task

Indulge yourself with new skincare items that you've been needing to attempt and another sack to keep them in that you're eager to utilize!

The easily overlooked details have a significant effect, and I guarantee, in the event that you adhere to a skincare routine reliably, you'll be stunned at the progressions you'll see!

Chapter 3: Embracing Different Skin Types

Each complexion is important and alluring and merits a similar consideration. At the point when we can acknowledge outside things, similar to the variety and kind of our skin, we'll have the option to acknowledge the more profound things - like our shortcomings and blemishes.

Before you discuss embracing different skin type you need to know your skin, right off the bat, types.

- **Identify and understanding various skin types**

What are various kinds of skin?

It could intrigue you to realize that there are various kinds of skin and each skin type requires a customized skincare routine. Also, while you and your companion could have a similar skin type, the circumstances can in any case vary as certain items that suit you probably won't suit the other individual.

This is to say that it is fundamental to decide your skin type and deal with it in manners that are the most ideal for that specific skin type to accomplish fast and wanted results. For the most part, there are five unique kinds of skin, and these skin types names are - Normal Skin, oily Skin, Dry Skin,combination Skin and sensitive Skin.

All unique skin types have various qualities. We should investigate these qualities:

Ordinary Skin
Ordinary skin is neither too dry nor excessively sleek and has a reasonable creation of sebum (regular skin oils) and

excess blood course. Normal skin is called normal skin as it has the ideal measure of sebum and doesn't experience the ill issues like skin inflammation or awareness.

Oily Skin

Oily skin delivers an oily encounter as your skin is creating a lot of sebum levels and that oil makes a layer all over. Individuals with slick skin will generally experience the ill effects of skin issues like skin break out breakouts and require additional consideration.

Dry Skin

Dry skin is one of the different skin types and is exceptionally normal in individuals living in dry natural circumstances. On the off chance that you have dry skin, your skin can become flaky and obtain an unpleasant surface. Because of dryness, your skin could try and turn out to be tight and disturb you.

combination Skin

One of the most provoking sorts of skin to deal with is mix skin. This skin is one that is a blend of dry skin and oily skin. While your T-zone (the region from the center of your eyebrows to the curves of the nose) can be oily , your cheeks and brow may be dry in this skin type.

Sensitive Skin

It is difficult to depict sensitive skin type by visual cues. Nevertheless, you may have fragile skin if you are prone to redness and irritation on your skin, especially after using new skincare products or after consuming hot meals.

Now that you know the various sorts of skin, the following stage is to respond to your inquiry 'How to realize my skin type?' There are various ways of finding out about your skin type by noticing the general wellbeing and sebum creation. Notwithstanding, to turn out to be certain beyond a shadow of doubt, you can attempt these strategies:

The bare-faced approach

Makeup remover should be used to remove all traces of makeup from your face.

Cleanse your face thoroughly with a gentle cleanser and pat dry softly. Allow your skin to restore to its natural state without using any products.

Check your face for oily traces after a while after washing it. keep an eye on the T zone

Result

Normal skin is free of oiliness and should feel smooth.

Oily skin has grease on it and appears shiny and silky to the touch. It is acne-prone and has big pores. It is critical to moisturize.

Combination skin is the most prevalent, with traces of all three skin types mentioned above. Typically, the skin has an oily T zone (forehead, nose, and chin) and normal skin everywhere else.

Sensitive skin is defined as a range of reactive skin problems that occur when the skin comes into contact with an allergen, producing irritation and triggering inflammation.

The blotting sheet approach:

This method is more faster and frequently provides a great distinction between oily and dry skin types. Gently pat a blotter paper on the different regions of your face, 39 minutes after washing your skin in the morning, and bring the sheet up to the light to see how much oil is visible.

-If the sheet absorbed little to no oil, you probably have dry skin.
-If the sheet displays oil from the brow and nose, your skin type is normal/combination.
-If the blotting paper is saturated with oil, you probably have oily skin.

How To Recognize Each Skin Type And Deal with Them?

Since you have a response to the inquiry 'What is my skin type?' We should sort out the best skincare routine for your skin type.

Normal skin type

In the event that you are honored with an ordinary skin type, you shouldn't underestimate it. Ordinary skin type implies that your skin's oil creation and pH are adjusted, and you are not inclined to skin issues like skin break out. By and large, a typical skin type doesn't need a point by point skincare schedule, however that doesn't mean you shouldn't deal with it. Here are ordinary and simple to follow tips that you can play out each day.

Use sunscreens both inside and outside as you can be presented to UV light even in your home through windows and devices. Use sunscreen with SPF 30 to keep a characteristic equilibrium.

Saturate your skin routinely and keep it hydrated by drinking water and utilizing toners.

Utilize advantageous fixings like L-ascorbic acid and E, regular concentrates, and so on, to keep up with your normal sparkle.

Eliminate your cosmetics consistently prior to nodding off to unclog your pores.

Oily skin type

Oily skin can occur because of a few reasons, which incorporate hereditary issues, hormonal changes, climatic changes, and so forth. As slick skin is more inclined to skin inflammation, you need to deal with it more. Follow these means in the event that you have a slick skin type.

Wash your skin with cleaners that retain oil and follow with a light lotion.

Use items with fixings, for example, salicylic corrosive and glycolic corrosive, in the event that you have skin break out.

Use water based, silicon based and gel based items to keep up with your sleek skin.

Don't over wash your skin or skip lotion, as it can prompt more sebum creation.

To degrease your face in a split second, use rice papers or blotching papers.

Dry skin type

the most effective method to realize skin type Dry skin is one of the most dangerous skin types as it can cause tingling, bothering, aggravation and dying. In the event that you have a dry skin type, you can follow these tips to deal with your skin.

The main thing is to saturate your skin two times every day.
Abstain from washing up as they can take regular oils from your face.
Utilize a humidifier in the event that you live in a dry region to keep your skin hydrated.
Search for items with fixings like mineral oil, zinc oxide, glycerin, squalene, olive oil, coconut oil, and so on.

Combination skin type

Having a combination skin type can be disappointing as certain districts of your face are sleek/oily and others dry. In the event that you have a mix skin type, these tips can take care of you.

Utilize a delicate product to try not to over animated bigger skin pores in T zone.

Have a go at utilizing two skincare schedules, one appropriate for sleek skin on T zone and one appropriate for dry skin on cheeks and brow.

By and large, don't involve items with oil as it would cause overabundance sebum emission from your T-zone.

Sensitive skin type

Sensitive skin by and large occurs because of the over responsiveness of sensitive spots present underneath your skin. It very well may be difficult to have delicate skin as it is effectively invigorated by outside factors. The following are a couple of tips to remember.

Counsel a dermatologist to sort out the right skincare items for your skin's pH balance.

Utilize a slim and lightweight cream.

Try not to utilize items with counterfeit scents, colors, parabens, and so forth.

Try not to utilize alcoholic toners and astringents.

Keep your body's nutrient and mineral levels at inferior with your body's prerequisite to give insusceptibility against aggravations.

One more significant thing to recall whether you have a delicate skin type or some other skin type is just to utilize regular healthy skin items that contain no synthetic compounds, parabens, or sulfates. You can depend on brands, for example, Unadulterated Sense, which offer a scope of skincare items produced using regular concentrates with no synthetic substances or poisons.

- ## Tailoring your skincare routine to your skin type

Having solid skin care routine, it is wanted by a larger number of people to gleam skin. However, little do individuals have at least some idea that the key to accomplishing that objective is to have a skincare schedule that works. Preparing a skincare schedule that will provide you with the skin of your fantasies may not necessarily be basically as straightforward as it sounds. You should think about a great deal of factors, and there are many items out there.

In any case, no problem, we've arranged this manual for assist with setting you in order. Simply don't surrender when you don't get results immediately. Remember that items will require some investment to do something amazing.

The different skin types

A skincare routine will fluctuate from one individual to a nother in light of the fact that each sort of skin is one of a kind. That is the reason before we bounce into the different skin regimens, you should initially decide your skin type so you can address your skin concerns enough.

There are five distinct kinds of skin;

normal,   Dry,oily,combination, and sensitive. By and large, one gains skin type through hereditary qualities. Yet, it might in any case change all through your lifetime, as different variables will influence your skin. Things like eating regimen, way of life, age, the environment of the locale where you live, and that's only the tip of the iceberg.

Do you have any idea what sort of skin you have? Peruse beneath to find out!

Ordinary/ normal

Ordinary skin types have the right harmony between dampness and sebum (the body's normal oils) creation in the skin. This kind of skin is less inclined to break out or experience the ill effects of skin conditions.

Normal indications of ordinary skin:

Pores are not excessively apparent

Liberated from flaws
Skin has a smooth surface
Not inclined to awareness
Neither excessively slick or excessively dry

DRY

Dry skin types produce deficient dampness and regular oil in the skin. It needs Regular Saturating Variables (NMFs) which draw in and tie water to the skin.

Normal indications of dry skin:

Skin feels tight and unpleasant
Skin is scaling, chipping, or feels irritated
The tone of the skin looks dull and smudged

Pores are not excessively apparent

Skin is inclined to drying and breaking

Sleek/oil

This kind of skin creates an abundance of sebum. It very well may be set off by factors like hereditary qualities, stress, hormonal unevenness, or prescription. Commonly, sleek skin types will have stopped up or blocked pores, making it inclined to issues like skin break out.

Normal indications of sleek skin:

Pores are enormous and apparent
Skin is glossy or looks oily
Skin looks stout and thick

Blend/combination

A blend skin type implies having sleek skin in a specific piece of the face and dry skin in one more piece of the face.

Normal indications of mix skin:

Slick T zone region
Dryness in cheeks
Expanded pores in the T zone region
Touchy

Delicate/sensitive

Delicate skin types are inclined to aggravation, bothering, stinging and consuming. This skin type can likewise have a brutal response to specific fixings. However, with most delicate skin, utilizing the right items can assist with settling the normal issues related with this skin type.

Normal indications of sensitive skin:

Redness
Consuming sensation on the skin
Skin feels dry and irritated

Acne prone/Skin break out Inclined

This kind of skin has a proclivity to create comedones and pimples. Skin break out or Skin break out Vulgaris, is a non-infectious skin condition brought about by the irritation and contamination of the sebaceous organs in the skin. Albeit generally normal among youths, a few side effects might endure into adulthood.

Normal indications of skin inflammation inclined skin:

Sleek and sparkling skin
Little, red, and delicate knots (papules) underneath the skin's surface
Papules with discharge at the tip (pustules)

Huge, strong, and excruciating knocks (knobs)

Normally shows up in the face, neck, shoulders, back, and chest

A Manual for SKINCARE Items

Presently it is the ideal time to be taught about healthy skin items. The sorts of items you put all over will influence the general wellbeing and state of your skin.

In the event that you've at any point been overpowered by the various types of skincare items on the lookout, here's an aide on the necessities you ought to be aware and be utilizing.

Cleanser

Purifying is the most basic move toward really focusing on the skin - this is non-debatable. The right cleanser shouldn't strip your skin of regular oils yet ought to help with eliminating the soil, impacts of air contamination, and overabundance sebum right in front of you. In this manner, leaving it entirely spotless and prepared for the subsequent stages.

Stay away from cleanser with sodium lauryl sulfate (SLS), sodium lauryl ether sulfate (SLES), aromas, and fragrances. In the event that your skin encounters stinging, snugness, or dryness in the wake of purging, select a delicate or hydrating cleaning agent rather than a slick skin chemical. Likewise, in the event that your skin turns out to be too oily inside a brief time frame in the wake of purifying, decide on a more grounded gel cleaning agent to clean your skin.

TONER

Utilizing toners will prepare the skin, so it obtains the most ideal outcomes from skincare items. It permits the skin to successfully ingest items more. Furthermore, toners assist with adjusting the pH level of the skin, and a pH-adjusted skin implies sound skin.

You can apply your toner by dousing a cotton cushion and skimming it across your face tenderly. You may likewise spread your toner on the centers of your hands then, at that point, pat it onto your skin. Forestall aggravating your skin by keeping away from toners that contain liquor and aromas.

SERUM

Serums contain strong and concentrated fixings that assist with focusing on unambiguous skin concerns. It is comprised of little particles that sink profound into the skin.

To apply serums, just delicately tap it onto your skin's trouble spots.

LOTION

All skin types benefit from lotions. This item secures in dampness and permits hydration into the skin. It additionally supports, smoothen, and full the skin.

Check the fixing rundown of your lotion, stay away from creams with counterfeit scents, colors, parabens, or phthalates.

SUNSCREEN

Sunscreen safeguards the skin from harm against hurtful UV

beams, untimely maturing, and even skin disease, making it a fundamental item in your skincare routine.

The most well-known synthetic substances found in sunscreens are Oxybenzone, Retinyl Palmitate, and Parabens. Oxybenzone retains UVA and UVB beams, while Retinyl Palmitate is a type of Vitamin A for skin break out. Both safeguard the skin from the destructive impacts of the sun and no realized investigations have inferred that both of these substances is carcinogenic

Nonetheless, a couple of studies propose that Parabens, which are additives utilized in numerous corrective items like sunscreens, behave like estrogen in the body, which can hurry the development of bosom disease growths. More probable, however, researchers accept that individuals who use sunscreens most are similar individuals who open themselves to the sun on a more regular basis, and may not be utilizing it appropriately, thus, the more serious gamble.

Sunscreen (ideally SPF 30 or higher) ought to be applied day to day, something like 20 minutes prior to going outside even on an overcast day. These days, in any event, when inside, our skin can in any case be presented to UV beams and blue light from devices like cell phones, workstations, and PCs. A definite approach to safeguarding your skin is by wearing sunscreen.

Extra NOTE:

With items, consistency is fundamental. It requires no less than about a month and a half to get results. Give close consideration to the progressions in your skin, check how your skin responds to the items then change your routine likewise. Additionally, NEVER apply items to your face when you have messy hands.

EVERYDAY SKINCARE ROUTINE FOR ORDINARY SKIN TYPES

As referenced, ordinary skin types are even. Support for this skin type is as yet fundamental, however, to constantly keep the skin sound and brilliant.

STAR Fixings

The fixings that work best with this skin type are Niacinamide, Green Tea, L-ascorbic acid, Vitamin E, Glycerin, Hyaluronic Corrosive, Aloe, Organic product, and Flower separates.

AM Normal

Scrub skin with a gentle frothing chemical or any water-based cleaning agent. Then, at that point, tone skin with a strong cell reinforcement like Coenzyme Q10. Subsequent to conditioning, apply a light-weight moisturizer. Then, at that point, apply a layer of sun insurance.

Tip: Spritz your face with rose water or a facial fog over the course of the day to perk up the vibe of your skin.

PM Schedule

Purge skin with a non-drying velvety facial cleaning agent. Apply your toner while your skin is still a piece clammy. Then, at that point, utilize a cell reinforcement serum like L-ascorbic acid to assist with fixing your skin. Polish off with a smooth cream.

EVERYDAY SKINCARE ROUTINE FOR DRY SKIN TYPES

For dry skin types, dampness and hydration are genuinely necessary for their consideration.

STAR Fixings

The fixings that work best with this skin type are Non-fragrant plant oils. Instances of these are Argan Oil, Marula Oil, and Night Primrose Oil, as well as Glycolic acid, Lactic acid, Hyaluronic Corrosive, and Ceramides.

AM Normal

Purge with tepid or cold water just, as high temp water strips the skin of regular oils, further drying your skin. Search for a delicate, hydrating cleaning agent to clean your face, or you might consider involving a micellar water answer for a no-flush choice.

In the wake of purging, it's crucial for utilize a liquor free toner to keep your skin from evaporating significantly more. Then utilize a hydrating, water-based serum and lotion to keep your skin from looking dull. Get done with a layer of sunscreen.

PM Schedule

Utilize delicate, hydrating purifying milk or cream-based cleaning agent with facial oils to clean and support the skin. Then keep your skin clammy by applying an emollient-based toner. It is ideal to utilize your toner on skin that is still a piece moist for better ingestion.

Keep on applying your serum, ideally one with a concentrated hyaluronic corrosive serum to forestall dampness misfortune while you rest. You may likewise pick to apply facial oil after your serum to support skin brilliance and hydration. Then, at that point, seal all items with a rich cream.

Tip: When the weather conditions is cold, and the stickiness is low, your skin is more inclined to aggravation, redness, and dryness because of the absence of dampness. Consider putting resources into a humidifier to add dampness out of sight and your skin.

Day to day skincare routine for oily skin typesKeep oil under control and forestall oily looking skin. Your objective ought to be to adjust your skin and not dry it out.

STAR Fixings

The fixings that work best with this skin type are Witch Hazel Concentrate, Tea Tree Oil, Ginseng, Rosehip, Salicylic acid, and Glycolic acid.

AM Standard

Purifying is crucial for individuals with slick skin since oil develops rapidly in the skin. Settle on a gel based or froth chemical to keep your skin clean. What's more, in the event that you are experiencing skin break out, search for a chemical with antibacterial properties like tea tree to assist with combatting skin break out.

In the wake of cleaning, rebalance your skin's pH level with a reviving toner then utilize a lightweight, water based cream. Search for a saturating item that is sans oil and non comedogenic. Obviously, remember to put on sunscreen.

PM Schedule

Assuming you regularly wear make-up, it is suggested that you clean your face two times around evening time. Twofold purifying is a notable technique for cleaning your face with an oil based chemical first then with a water-based cleaning agent second.

Then utilize a toner with fixings like AHA or BHA so it can enter profound into your pores and eliminate the leftover overabundance oil and soil from your face. Then hydrate your skin with a lotion.

Tip: Peel in the wake of purging on more than one occasion per week to quagmire off dead skin and keep pores from being stopped up and blocked.

DAT TO DAY SKINCARE ROUTINE FOR

COMBINATION SKIN TYPES

Really focusing on a blend skin type might be a piece interesting as certain region of the face are dry while different regions are sleek. However, with a touch of persistence, your skin can look comparable, as well.

STAR Fixings

The fixings that work best with this skin type are Lactic acid, Green Tea, Aloe Vera, Honey, Calendula, and Hyaluronic acid.

AM Standard

A gentle, smooth cleaning agent or micellar water functions admirably on this skin type. You ought to then adjust the pH level of your skin with a liquor free toner. Follow it up with a cell reinforcement serum, a lightweight water cream lotion, and sunscreen.

PM Schedule

Purify skin with a gentle, cream based chemical. Peeling on more than one occasion week by week is discretionary yet suggested. Subsequent to purifying, apply a liquor free toner. Make certain to try not to apply a toner with witch hazel or tea tree on the dry pieces of your face.

Tenderly search your face with a rich serum, ideally, one that contains hyaluronic corrosive. Then, at that point, apply a weighty emollient lotion on the dry pieces of your face and light, gel cream put together cream with respect to the sleek pieces of your face.

Tip: Attempt multi veiling on more than one occasion per week to add gleam to your skin. Multi-concealing means applying various kinds of facial coverings to various region of your face to address different skin worries simultaneously.

DAY TO DAY SKINCARE ROUTINE FOR SENSITIVE SKIN TYPES

Sensitive skin needs exceptional consideration, really take a look at the rundown of fixings in the items and keep away from unforgiving synthetic substances, parabens, colors, and sulfates.

STAR Fixings

The fixings that work best with this skin type are Cereal, Aloe Vera, Cucumber, Chamomile, and Rice Concentrate.

AM Normal

Find an unscented or cleanser free chemical to use in the first part of the day to clean and revive your skin, then, at that point, mitigate skin with a delicate toner. Hydrate your skin with a light cream then finish it off with sunscreen. Mineral sunscreen works best with this sort of skin.

PM Schedule

Utilize a delicate purifying cream, gel or oil that will successfully eliminate your cosmetics as well as perfect your face.

Verify whether your skin can endure any serums with acids like mandelic acid. Gradually bring the acid into your skin first. In the event that your skin responds well to it, use it no less than two times every week. Then, at that point, utilize a gel or water based lotion to seal in dampness unto your skin.

Tip: Stay away from compound sunscreen and physical exfoliants. Go for scent free items with basic fixings to diminish the possibilities having a hypersensitive response to the item.

EVERYDAY SKINCARE ROUTINE FOR SKIN BREAKOUT INCLUDED SKIN TYPES

A few factors like hormonal skin inflammation changes during pubescence and pregnancy, climatic area (warm and damp environments), and, surprisingly, the utilization of specific medicine and beauty care products can set off the breakout of skin inflammation. It is particularly essential to embrace an everyday healthy skin routine in the event that your skin is inclined to skin inflammation.

STAR Fixings

The best fixings to address skin inflammation inclined skin are Salicylic Acid, Vitamin A and C, Shedding Granules, Hyaluronic acid, Kaolin Dirt, and Benzoyl Peroxide.

AM Standard

Utilize your fingertips or a delicate washcloth to wash your skin completely. Utilize a gel or froth based cleaning agent that is non comedogenic, non allergenic, and non crabby. These items can eliminate soil yet at the same time keep the skin from being harmed.

Utilize a cotton ball or smooth cushion to apply toner to your face and neck to assist with eliminating oil, cosmetics, and chemical deposits as well as hydrate and forestall skin imperfections. Try to utilize toners that don't dry out your skin.

Smooth on your endorsed or over-the-counter skin break out

treatment creams. Ensure your face is completely spotless and dry prior to applying your creams. Likewise, let your skin retain the drug prior to continuing to the subsequent stage.

Some hormonal skin break out prescriptions might dry out skin, so it is essential to apply without oil and non-comedogenic saturating gels or salves to keep the skin from drying or stripping.

PM Schedule

In the event that you wear cosmetics during the day or your day's exercises (like broad exercises or sports) make you sweat vigorously, do a twofold wash around evening time. That implies purge, wash well, then, at that point, rehash. Doing this will ensure all the cosmetics, soil, and sweat are washed away consistently.

Apply toner all over and neck following similar headings in the first part of the day schedule.

Apply your endorsed or over-the-counter skin break out treatment creams following similar bearings in the first part of the day schedule.

Saturate your skin with a sans oil and non comedogenic saturating moisturizer.

THE SIGNIFICANT OF HAVING A LEGITIMATE SKINCARE SCHEDULE

Various kinds of skin require interesting consideration. Regardless of whether an item is known to be extraordinary and groundbreaking, you probably won't see as phenomenal an outcome in the event that it's not implied for your facial sort. In addition to the fact that that is a misuse of cash and exertion you could hurt your skin that way.

There isn't one skincare schedule that fits a wide range of skin. These regimens are to be changed by your singular requirements. So having a legitimate skincare routine guarantees that your skin stays sound by getting the right items and medicines.

Chapter 4: Common facial Skin Problems

Taking proper care of your skin is a job. Aside from simply remembering to complete your twice-a-day skin care routine, there are a plethora of skin concerns .some are-:

1. pigmentation

2. Pores

3. Dark circle

4. Acne

5. wrinkle

6. uneven skin

7. Brown spot

8. Scars

9. Dull skin

10. Black head

11. White head

12. papules

13. Pustules and others.

- **Type of acid in Skincare and their benefit:**

How do acids help your skin?

Face acids are exfoliants. They work to turn over layers of dead skin cells faster than would occur all alone. That implies facial acids can assist with making your skin smoother and more brilliant. They assist with battling skin break out. Furthermore, they forestall and switch the harm that prompts issues like redness, age spots and kinks.

There are two principal sorts of acids utilized in skin health management:

Alpha hydroxy acids (AHAs) are water-solvent acids. They slacken the liquid that ties surface skin cells together. That permits dead skin cells to swamp off. "As we age, the paste that keeps our skin cells intact becomes denser, which dials back the normal

cell turnover process," Stein makes sense of. "AHAs help to relax that paste and eliminate the dead cells that gunk up the top layer of our skin."
Beta hydroxy acids (BHAs) are oil-solvent acids. They enter further into your pores than AHAs. Like AHAs, BHAs assist remove with dead cleaning. Be that as it may, they likewise assist with dissolving sebum, a slick substance your body makes. Overabundance sebum can prompt skin inflammation.
In any case, not all skin health management acids fall into these classes. Favoring that in a little.

The significant thing to recall pretty much all face acids is that their responsibility is to peel, and you would rather not overdo it.

"To a degree, shedding can be something to be thankful for. Yet, a lot of can likewise be disturbing in light of the fact that you're basically stripping the top layer of your skin," Stein states. "Face acids can be perfect to assist with working on your skin's surface, even out staining and different advantages, however you would rather not strip it such a lot of that you eliminate the great pieces of the skin, similar to the designs that hold in water and sound fats."

Something else to recollect: Utilizing facial acids can result in you more inclined to sun harm. That is on the grounds that acids uncover sound, new cells that are more vulnerable to the sun. Thus, Stein says it's crucial to utilize SPF 30 (or higher) sunscreen all over each day. Sunscreen will assist with safeguarding you from sun related burn, skin disease and the maturing impacts of the sun's beams.

a portion of the more normal face acids and how they work.

1. Salicylic acid

Salicylic acid is a Beta Hydroxy corrosive known for its capacity to diminish skin inflammation on the skin. It assists with shedding the skin at a cell level by entering the skin layers and dissolving the dead skin cells. It additionally helps in unclogging the blocked pores and obstructed hair follicles by clearing the overabundance sebum, amassed soil, and grime. This activity, thus, helps in lessening zits and whiteheads, together named as non-fiery skin break out.

In a higher fixation, salicylic acid goes about as a stripping specialist and is many times used to treat skin break out, skin break out scars, melasma, and age spots. Notwithstanding, there are a few secondary effects that you can anticipate from utilizing salicylic acid. However generally protected on the skin, abuse of salicylic acid can cause skin aggravation or outrageous dryness. You could encounter stripping of the skin in the initial not many days after you begin utilizing the acid. Notwithstanding, easily affected responses are rare, and you are generally going to partake in the sensation of smooth skin on utilizing it.

2. Glycolic acid

Glycolic acid is an Alpha Hydroxy acid that is gotten from sugarcane. This fixing also assists in treating with cleaning breakouts and skin inflammation. Glycolic acid, when topically applied, enters the skin and breaks the desmosomal connections between the shallow epidermal layer and the fundamental dermal layers. This activity strips off the external skin layer and assists you with wiping out the solidified, dull and dead skin cells, and uncovers smoother and more splendid skin.

Glycolic acid likewise helps in holding dampness in the skin cells and forestalls drying out the skin. Research has shown it to have antibacterial as well as cancer prevention agent properties. Glycolic acid even aides improve collagen combination, which thickens the skin and makes it more grounded and more versatile.

3. Ascorbic acid

Ascorbic acid, otherwise called L-ascorbic acid, is one more intense facial acid with different skin benefits. It is a rich wellspring of cell reinforcements and forestalls free extremists on the skin. This forestalls skin harm and postpones the maturing system. Ascorbic acid likewise advances collagen amalgamation, which makes the skin firmer and stronger.

L-ascorbic acid is additionally known to ease up the complexion by restraining the tyrosinase movement answerable for melanin (skin color) blend. It is likewise useful in forestalling indications of sun harm. One more advantage of this fixing is recharging Vitamin E supply in the skin, which shields the skin from sun harm.

4. Hyaluronic acid

Hyaluronic acid is another normally happening acid. Artificially talking, they are long unbranched chains of carbs or polysaccharides, known as glycosaminoglycans, present in our body's connective tissues. It gives our skin its design and uprightness. In any case, with propelling age, the HA present in our body actuates the presence of maturing signs. That is the point at which you want effective Hyaluronic acid.

HA is a strong humectant that attracts dampness from the environmental factors and keeps the skin very much hydrated. This, thus, builds the skin's flexibility, diminishes kinks and barely recognizable differences, and makes the skin delicate and graceful. It likewise helps in quicker p mending. Hyaluronic acid is utilized in dealing with skin problems like dermatitis as well.

5. Azelaic acid

Azelaic acid is a natural corrosive got from grains like grain, wheat, and rye. It is well known for its antimicrobial and calming properties, which assist with dealing with skin conditions like skin inflammation and rosacea. It helps keep skin inflammation causing microscopic organisms under control by getting out the open pores. It likewise upgrades the phone turnover rate, helps with quicker twisted recuperating, and limits scarring.

Azelaic acid is likewise powerful in treating hyperpigmentation and disappears dim spots and fixes. Notwithstanding, it has a few incidental effects as well. One could encounter a consuming or shivering sensation, stripping and chipping of the skin, skin dryness, and redness. It could likewise make the skin flimsy and make it more delicate to sun harm.

6. Lactic acid

Lactic acid is one more Alpha hydroxy acid got from milk. It is viewed as a powerful enemy of maturing specialist as well as a pigmentation-battling fixing. Like a synthetic strip, this acid assists swamp off the evaporated external layer of the skin and raises the more splendid, more brilliant skin with layering under. It can assist with decreasing age spots and give your skin an even composition.

Lactic acid is a lot milder than most other AHAs and is in this manner facial acid of decision for touchy skin individuals. In any case, utilizing lactic acid can make your skin more helpless to sun harm. It could likewise cause skin disturbance, rash, and irritation, which generally dies down as the skin gets to know the fixing.Lactic acid strip isn't suggested assuming that you have a current skin condition like dermatitis, psoriasis, or rosacea.

7. Mandelic acid

Mandelic acid is a naturalacidc among the Alpha Hydroxy Acids acquired from unpleasant almonds. It is a milder acid reasonable for touchy skin. This acid can gradually get assimilated in the skin and speed up cell turnover by shedding the dead skin cells. It is likewise answerable for further developing collagen arrangement, in this manner making the skin solid and versatile.

Mandelic acid is likewise useful in treating skin inflammation and breakouts by directing sebum creation and unclogging pores. It likewise has a calming activity that lessens pimples and flaws. It makes the skin smoother by eliminating the dull and evaporated skin cells stored in the shallow layers and uncovering the more brilliant layer under. A similar activity likewise helps in disappearing hyperpigmentation.

By advancing collagen creation, mandelic acid likewise diminishes kinks and barely recognizable differences and gives your skin a young appearance.

8. Ferulic acid

Ferulic acid is gotten from different sources like grain, oats, rice, eggplants, and even citrus natural products. Likewise a rich wellspring of cell reinforcements battle against the free extremists in the skin. It even lifts the presentation of different cell reinforcements like L-ascorbic acid, An and E. It additionally assists with settling L-ascorbic acid and offers assurance against sun harm.

It has been demonstrated to diminish the gamble of skin malignant growth too successfully. It is generally protected on the skin however could cause extremely touchy responses in specific individuals. An aversion to ferulic acid can encounter redness, rashes, hives, irritation, and in any event, stripping and chipping of the skin.

9. Kojic acid

Kojic acid is gotten from different parasites types, predominantly by maturing food sources like Japanese purpose, soy sauce, and rice wine. It is most famous in view of its magnificent skin-easing up properties. It restrains tyrosine (an amino acid liable for melanin union) arrangement and lessens skin hyperpigmentation.

Kojic acid likewise helps in fending off a few microbes and lessens skin break out somewhat. It additionally has against contagious properties that assist with treating different skin contaminations. It very well may be utilized to deal with conditions like candidiasis, ringworm, or competitor's foot. However typically protected on the skin, involving in lower concentrations is best. Kojic acid could cause contact dermatitis and lead to skin aggravation, redness, irritation, rashes, and enlarging.

10.Malic acid

Malic acid is ordered under Alpha Hydroxy acids. This corrosive is gotten from squeezed apple and sheds dull shallow skin. It further develops cell recovery and gives the skin an energetic appearance. Being a humectant, it attracts dampness from the climate, improves skin hydration, diminishes kinks, and leaves your skin a smoother surface. Malic acid additionally helps in adjusting pH levels. Malic acid likewise assumes a part in easing up skin break out scars .It eliminates abundance oil and soil from the skin and forestalls skin break out.

A few Less popular Acids With Extraordinary Advantages

Linoleic acid: Known for pigmentation easing up capacity.
Oleic acid: Goes about as a transporter that assists in shipping different

medications by entering the skin with layering.

Lipoic acid: Has a high measure of cell reinforcements and furthermore helps in postponing maturing.

Alguronic acid: Goes about as an enemy of maturing specialist.

The Main concern:

Subsequent to perusing this article, we genuinely trust you will pick acids to cure your skin burdens. To make things simple for you somewhat more, here's the concise variant of the useful impacts of the different facial acids initially.

Hyaluronic acid is quite possibly of the most powerful humectant that can assist in keeping the skin with welling saturated.

Battling against skin break out, salicylic acid, glycolic acid acid acid, mandelic acid, lactic acid, and azelaic acid can help.

Ascorbic acid, lactic acid, glycolic acid, and ferulic acid can be superb solutions for fix maturing signs. They can cause your skin to show up more brilliant and young.

You can incorporate kojic acid, lactic acid, ascorbic acid, linoleic acid, or even ferulic acid in your skincare system for treating hyperpigmentation.

● Different ingredients in skincare and their benefit

1. Parabens

Parabens are a group of synthetic additives originally presented during the 1950s. They're utilized to drag out time span of usability in many preparing items by forestalling mold and microbes development inside them.

They've been connected to malignant growth and chemical interruption. Parabens can likewise sharpen the skin, causing hypersensitive responses.

You can find Parabens in shampoos, conditioners, body washes, and lotions.

Parabens are recorded as:

methylparaben
propylparaben
butylparaben
thylparaben.

2. Phthalates

Phthalates are boring, unscented, sleek synthetic compounds added to plastic to stop it becoming fragile.

They are likewise utilized as gelling specialists (they assist with blending fixings that wouldn't typically blend) in certain shampoos and in other prepping items to assist them with adhering to your skin.

They've been connected to birth imperfections and chemical disturbance and are being checked by the FDA.

Phlalates are recorded as:

diethylphthalate
monoethyl

3. Formaldehyde

Indeed - a similar stuff used to protect carcasses is likewise utilized in a scope of prepping items to assist with keeping them new by forestalling microbiological development.

Formaldehyde has solid connects to asthma, neurotoxicity, disease, and formative poisonousness.

Formaldehyde is recorded as:

formic aldehyde
methanethiol

4. Scent/Parfum

"Scent" is an umbrella term. It could mean a blend of allergens, cancer-causing agents, or aggravations.

The name 'Scent' or 'Parfum' was created to safeguard an organization's proprietary innovations under the Fair Bundling and Marking Demonstration of 1966.

Aroma/Parfum is recorded as:

aroma

parfums

Assuming you're searching for a cream that is liberated from counterfeit scent, saturates your face well and won't create any disturbances, look at our regular Face Lotion.

5. Mineral oil

Mineral oil is an unmistakable, scentless fluid that has been utilized regularly for a long time in a wide assortment of prepping items. It is modest, scent free, and dreary, doesn't oxidize, and can without much of a stretch be saved for quite a while - making it extremely famous in the prepping business.

Mineral oil is an occlusive emollient, implying that it assists with keeping your skin hydrated by securing in dampness by framing an obstruction on your skin's surface.

Openness to mineral oils is unequivocally connected with an expanded gamble of nonmelanoma skin malignant growth, especially the scrotum.

Mineral oil is recorded as:

paraffinum liquidum
petrolatum
cera microcristallina
microcrystalline wax
ozokerite
ceresin paraffin
paraffin
manufactured wax

6. Butylated Hydroxytoluene (BHT)

BHT is a manufactured additive that upsets chemicals, prompts hypersensitive responses, and disturbs testosterone levels.

Long haul openness to high portions of BHT causes liver, thyroid, and kidney issues in mice.

You can track down BHT in creams, antiperspirants, and exfoliators.

BHT is recorded as:
BHT

7. Aluminum

Aluminum is a typical fixing in antiperspirants. The aluminum intensifies found in antiperspirants lessen sweat by hindering your underarm perspiration channels.

It additionally limits stench by restraining the scent delivering microbes that feed on your perspiration.

A few investigations show that individuals presented to high aluminum levels might foster Alzheimer's infection.

Aluminum is recorded as:
aluminum
aluminum zirconium
tetrachlorohydrex GLY
aluminum chlorohydrate
To view as a characteristic, without aluminum antiperspirant that scents astounding, look at our Normal Antiperspirant - Sea.

8. Coal tar colors

Coal tar is a combination of numerous synthetic substances that come from petrol. It fills a viable need in the 1

You can recognize coal tar color by a five-digit Variety File (CI) number

The US variety name may likewise be recorded ("FD&C" or "D&C" trailed by a variety name and number)

9. Stake compounds

Stakes (polyethylene glycols) are oil based intensifies utilized in preparing items as thickeners, solvents, conditioners, and dampness transporters.

Assuming utilized on broken or harmed skin, Stakes can cause disturbance and framework poisonousness. Stakes can decrease the skin's dampness levels and accelerate skin maturing.

Stake compounds are recorded as:

poly(ethylene oxide)
poly(oxyethylene).

10. Siloxanes

Siloxanes make hair items dry rapidly and they cause creams to apply all the more easily. Siloxanes have been displayed to slow down human chemical capability.

Siloxanes are recorded as:

Cyclopentasiloxane

11. Triclosan

The corrective business utilizes triclosan as an additive to prevent microbes from developing on the item and ruining it. It's a biocide (an item that controls destructive or undesirable life forms through synthetic or natural means) in numerous other individual consideration items like antiperspirants, cleansers, and shower gels.

It firmly associates with the debilitating of the invulnerable framework, uncontrolled cell development, and formative and regenerative harmfulness.

You can find them in antibacterial cleansers, antiperspirants, face washes, shower gels.

Triclosan is recorded as:

hydroxy diphenyl ether

microbeads in beauty care products harmful skincare fixing

12. Plastic microbeads

Microbeads are little, steady, produced plastic particles (made of polyethylene). They don't corrupt or disintegrate in water.

Body - Microbeads can enter the body through dermal assimilation. On the off chance that they get at you, they stall out under the eyelids and scratch the eyeballs. Proceeded with utilization of microbeads can prompt different contaminations because of the dabs causing scarring, departing your skin with scraped areas. Subsequently, miniature scarring can make your skin defenseless against bacterial assaults and different poisons, further focusing on your skin and accelerating the indications of maturing.

Climate - The pieces are sufficiently little to go through water filtration plants and hence end up in lakes and streams. You can find them in the Icy ocean ice and on the sea depths. A solitary shower can bring about 100,000 plastic particles entering the sea.

You'll find plastic microbeads in some face scours, body cleans and exfoliators

Plastic microbeads are recorded as:

polyethylene (PE),
polyethylene terephthalate (PET),
nylon (Dad),
polypropylene (PP),

polymethyl methacrylate (PMMA).
Outline

Recall this the following time you go out on the town to shop. Make a point to pause for a minute to concentrate on in the fixings rundown and reconsider snatching your 'go-to' cleanser, cream, or hair gel.

What Are Dynamic Fixings?

Dynamic fixings are utilized in skincare items to convey a few unique advantages for the client. They can be found in practically a wide range of skincare items right now available, and have become progressively well known for use in normal beauty care products.

Instances of dynamic fixings incorporate cancer prevention agents like Vitamin A, L-ascorbic acid and Vitamin E. Probiotics, Alpha-Hydroxy Corrosive (AHA), Hyaluronic Corrosive and Coenzyme Q10 are additionally well known dynamic elements for skincare items.

Abusing dynamic fixings can harm your skin, particularly on the face, where skin is more slender. You could cause more mischief than anything, for this reason it's especially vital to figure out dynamic fixings assuming that you are making Do-It-Yourself skincare items and to adhere to the suggested use rates. Utilizing more than the suggested most extreme rate doesn't build the advantages of the dynamic fixings, however will add pointless expenses for your detailing. The producers of the dynamic fixings have tried them completely to learn what sum works best and what finds a place with current guidelines.

When you have a comprehension of dynamic fixings and their singular advantages, it is feasible to make tailor-made skincare items appropriate for your skin type and any skin issues you might have, for example, dry, delicate or bad tempered skin, dermatitis inclined or skin inflammation inclined skin.

On the other hand, you could choose dynamic fixings that have more unambiguous capabilities, like assisting with decreasing the presence of almost negligible differences and kinks. Others can uphold the development of sebum (the slick, waxy substance normally created by your body). This will safeguard the skin from harm brought about by outside factors as well as from parchedness, subsequently keeping your skin super-hydrated and gleaming consistently.

Instances of Dynamic Fixings in Skincare and Their Advantages
a lady contacting her face in the wake of utilizing skincare items
The following is a rundown of dynamic fixings usually utilized in skincare items and the justification for why they are so well known. Kindly don't be put off by "corrosive", these are not brutal

or risky acids. Acids utilized in surface level items are utilized at such low focuses that they represent no serious danger to your skin or wellbeing.

Alpha-Hydroxyacid (AHA) - The Exfoliator
Shedding is crucial for assist with eliminating soil and oil trapped in your skin's pores. A great many people utilize grating physical exfoliators that incorporate Apricot Piece Powder or Jojoba Peeling Grains. In any case, those with exceptionally delicate skin ought to know not to abuse such materials as their skin might respond to an excess of peeling.

All things considered, AHA can be utilized to do a similar occupation without the actual cleaning of your skin. AHA is a synthetic exfoliator (not quite as terrifying as it sounds) that assists with releasing dead skin cells, soil, and oil with no scouring at all. AHA leaves your skin spotless, hydrated and feeling smooth and prepared for saturating.

AHA's come in various structures, including glycolic, lactic and mandelic acids. All are ok for use on delicate skin, when utilized at the right rates, yet ought not be applied to dried out or open skin. Aromantic's AHA's are a blend of regular natural product extricates found in blueberries, sugar stick, oranges, lemons, and sugar maple.

Hyaluronic acid - The Super-Hydrator

Hyaluronic acid (HA) has become very famous throughout recent years for its capacity to assimilate and hold dampness inside the skin. HA is most popular for holding up to multiple times its weight in water, and that implies it pulls water to your skin like no other fixing available. The outcome? Very hydrated skin.

Hyaluronic acid is normally delivered by your skin, yet the creation dials back fundamentally in your thirties. Applying a serum or cream including HA consistently will assist your skin with holding more dampness and take into consideration delicate, smooth, hydrated and solid looking skin.

Because of its hydrating properties, HA is a well known dynamic fixing among those with dry, mature and dermatitis inclined skin.

Some Hyaluronic acid available is creature obtained making it inadmissible for vegetarians and the people who wish to utilize brutality free items. Plant based HA's, for example, that sold by Aromantic is made utilizing a veggie lover reasonable maturation process.

L-ascorbic acid - The Brightener
Effective L-ascorbic acid contains cell reinforcements that can assist with

making your skin shine. It likewise battles against UV harm and works on the adequacy of sunscreens. Nonetheless, L-ascorbic acid is an interesting fixing that is inclined to insecurity. At Aromantic, we sell the steady type of restorative grade L-ascorbic acid , Sodium Ascorbyl Phosphate, which is great for use in skincare plans.

Vitamin E - The Defender
You might have seen that Vitamin E has been a famous fixing in skincare items for the overwhelming majority, numerous years. This is on the grounds that Vitamin E is a strong cell reinforcement that decreases harm by free revolutionaries, dials back oxidation in items, as well as being

very helpful in skincare items intended to lessen the presence of scarring. It can likewise assist with balancing out L-ascorbic acid (above). Vitamin E is normally tracked down on the skin, yet it is drained when presented to UV light. Adding a piece extra as a skin item will assist with supporting the skin's insurance from the sun's strong beams, however it ought not be mistaken for a sunscreen.

Vitamin A - The Cunning individual

You will presumably have caught wind of the "supernatural occurrence" fixing, retinol or Vitamin A. Frequently promoted just like the way to hostile to maturing, retinol is most usually utilized in lotions and serums that case to move back the years and make you look youthful once more. Retinol might assist with diminishing the presence of kinks, however it's anything but a marvel answer for maturing. As a matter of fact, abuse of retinol can deliver the skin more delicate to ecological aggressors and really accelerate maturing.

Aromantic stocks the steady type of Vitamin A, Retinyl Palmitate which is utilized in extremely low rates as it is so strong. Its strong cancer prevention agent properties help to safeguard cell layers from free extreme harm, animate skin cell reestablishment, support collagen creation and decrease the presence of almost negligible differences and kinks, bringing about apparently more youthful looking skin.

Also, it balances irritation and assists the skin with fixing itself, so is the ideal expansion to hostile to skin inflammation kind of items.

Niacinamide - The Aggravation Buster Aggravation of the skin is regularly brought about by ecological aggressors like contamination, stress, less than stellar eating routine and absence of rest. Those with dry or dermatitis inclined skin will be beyond what mindful of how irritation can assume control over your life.

While forestalling ecological aggressors can be testing, Niacinamide can assist with managing the eventual outcomes, including knocks, rashes and bothersome patches. Niacinamide is a subsidiary of Vitamin B3 and has regular mitigating and cell reinforcement properties. It can assist with lighting up the skin before sun-down out complexion and refine pores. On the off chance that you have extremely touchy skin, it will lessen your skin's responsiveness. Significantly more, is that it decreases TEWL (trans epidermal water misfortune) consequently further developing skin moisturisation, and supports the creation of normal emollients in the skin which all assistance to keep up with skin versatility keeping it looking sound.

Peptides - The Collagen Supporter
Regular peptides can assist with loosening up kinks and increment

collagen creation. This has made peptides a famous dynamic fixing around the world, and can be tracked down in numerous magnificence items that case to have hostile to maturing properties — However, they really do should be utilized at a decent working level to make a decent difference. Our Lupine Peptides are a mix of penta-and hexa-peptides that work as a MMP inhibitor. MMP represents Grid Metalloproteinase. MMP's activity is to debase proteins like collagen and elastin. These two are the characterizing elements of connective tissue, so remembering Lupine Peptides for your item builds the contractile limit of the fibroblast of the dermis, in this way decreasing the deficiency of immovability and versatility of the skin. There are guidelines on the site to guarantee you truly do utilize a decent and successful working level.

Utilize Lupine Peptides in blend with Hyaluronic acid Gel to full up the skin and lessen scarce differences and kinks.

Ceramides - The Hindrance Manufacturer

You might have heard various times that solid skin is the consequence of a sound skin boundary. One basic key to a sound skin hindrance is ceramides, which help to brace the boundary. Ceramides are lipids (unsaturated fats) that are found normally in the highest layers of the skin and in regular transporter oils. They do a very great job of keeping out contaminations and soil from your pores by shaping a defensive layer on your skin that limits dampness misfortune.

As we progress in years, our body's development of ceramides diminishes, so utilizing a cream with a decent equilibrium of transporter oils is a magnificent method for developing the ceramides in your skin's boundary and keep the skin hydrated.

Picking the Right Dynamic Elements for Your Skin
We as a whole have one of a kind skin that requires various degrees of care and consideration. Certain individuals are lucky and never need to stress over doing a lot for their skin. Be that as it

may, a significant number of us need to sustain and safeguard our skin to keep it solid and looking perfect.

Anyway, how would you pick the right dynamic elements for your skin? Here are some broad, however not authoritative, rules you can observe. You might need to do an experimentation examination to track down the best elements for your skin. Your skin is extraordinary, thus what works for one individual may not work for another.

Ordinary and oily Skin: Niacinamide and Retinol.
Dry Skin: Hyaluronic acid, Vitamin E and Ceramides.

Maturing: Lupine Peptides, Vitamin A, L-ascorbic acid and Vitamin E.

Pigmentation Issues: Hyaluronic acid, Vitamin B3 (Niacinamide) and L-ascorbic acid.

Bothered Skin: Vitamin A, Ceramides, Vitamin B3 (Niacinamide).

- ## Preventive measures for longterm skin health

Try not to possess energy for escalated skin health management? You can in any case spoil yourself by acing the fundamentals. Great skin health management and sound way of life decisions can assist with deferring regular maturing and forestall different skin issues. Begin with these five straightforward tips.

1. Shield yourself from the sun

One of the main ways of dealing with your skin is to shield it from the sun. A long period of sun openness can cause wrinkles, age spots and other skin issues — as well as increment the gamble of skin malignant growth.

For the absolute most complete sun assurance:

Use sunscreen. Utilize a wide range sunscreen with a SPF of something like 15. Apply sunscreen liberally, and reapply at regular intervals — or on a more regular basis in the event that you're swimming or sweating.

Look for conceal. Stay away from the sun between 10 a.m. what's more, 4 p.m., when the sun's beams are most grounded.

Wear defensive attire. Cover your skin with firmly woven long-sleeved shirts, long jeans and wide-overflowed caps. Likewise consider clothing added substances, which provide clothing with an extra layer of bright insurance for a specific number of washings, or unique sun-defensive dress — which is explicitly intended to obstruct bright beams.

2. Try not to smoke

Smoking makes your skin look more established and adds to wrinkles.

Smoking river the little veins in the furthest layers of skin, which diminishes blood stream and makes skin paler. This additionally exhausts the skin of oxygen and supplements that are mean a lot to skin wellbeing.

Smoking additionally harms collagen and elastin — the strands that invigorate your skin and flexibility. Likewise, the dreary looks you make while smoking —, for example, tightening your lips while breathing in and squinting your eyes to keep out smoke — can add to wrinkles.

Moreover, smoking expands your gamble of squamous cell skin malignant growth. Assuming you smoke, the most ideal way to safeguard your skin is to stopped. Ask your PCP for tips or medicines to assist you with halting smoking.

3. Treat your skin tenderly

Everyday purifying and shaving can negatively affect your skin. To keep it delicate:

Limit shower time. Heated water and long showers or showers eliminate oils from your skin. Limit your shower or shower time, and utilize warm — as opposed to hot — water.

Stay away areas of strength for from. Solid cleansers and cleansers can take oil from your skin. All things being equal, pick gentle chemicals.

Shave cautiously. To secure and grease up your skin, apply shaving cream, salve or gel prior to shaving. For the nearest shave, utilize a spotless, sharp razor. Shave toward the path the hair develops, not against it.

Wipe off. Subsequent to washing or washing, delicately pat or smudge your skin dry with a towel so some dampness stays on your skin.

Saturate dry skin. In the event that your skin is dry, utilize a lotion that accommodates your skin type. For everyday use, consider a lotion that contains SPF.

4. Eat a solid eating routine

A sound eating routine can help you look and feel your best. Eat a lot of natural products, vegetables, entire grains and lean proteins. The relationship among diet and skin inflammation isn't clear — however some exploration proposes that an eating regimen wealthy in fish oil or fish oil enhancements and low in undesirable fats and handled or refined carbs could advance more youthful looking skin. Drinking a lot of water helps keep your skin hydrated.

5. Oversee pressure

Uncontrolled pressure can make your skin more touchy and trigger skin inflammation breakouts and other skin issues. To support solid skin — and a sound perspective — do whatever it takes to deal with your pressure. Get sufficient rest, put forth sensible lines, downsize your daily agenda and make time to do the things you appreciate.

Chapter 5: Mastering Makeup Techniques

What goes first?
Knowing the Approaches to Apply Cosmetics.
Using Your Discretion to Purchase.Take You
Cosmetics Concentrate on a Higher
Level.Step-by-Step Guide to Leveling Up Your
Cosmetics Cycle Additionally
How Can Novices Buy Cosmetics?
Your Beauty Routine Significantly Improved.

● The correct order of makeup

1. The Best Technique for Applying Cream
2. The best way to use foundational knowledge
3. The best way to use fluid establishment
4. Detailed instructions for using concealer
5. Detailed directions for using establishment powder
6. Bronzer application technique that works the best
7. Blush application technique that works the best
8. Guidelines for Using a Highlighter
9. How to Apply Eyeshadow the Best Way
10. The Best Eyeliner Application Technique
11. How to Apply Mascara in the Best Way
12. The best technique for applying lip gloss
13. The Best Technique for Using Setting Spray

Stage 1: Lotion.
Woman putting lotion on her face

Give yourself enough time to prime your skin with a great lotion before you begin applying makeup. Choosing the appropriate kind of lotion is a crucial component of the puzzle. Let's look at the several types you may use, listed from lightest to heaviest:

Face fogs: This are water-based mixtures that may include certain nutrients and fragrances that are beneficial to the skin. While facial fogs aren't meant to replenish your skin's moisture content, they may be a helpful tool for maintaining a dewy appearance all day. Basically, spray whenever your skin feels dry over the day.

Serums: This are a thin layer of makeup that the skin absorbs efficiently. Numerous serums are available that are designed to specifically target certain pain locations. Certain serums help you hydrate your skin to prevent wrinkles, while other serums have ingredients that might brighten a dull complexion.

Salves: The most popular form of lotion is a cream, which works for a variety of skin types. Choose creams labeled as "non-comedogenic"; these products aim to prevent pore obstruction.

Creams: This can be the perfect time to invest in a cream lotion if you have dry skin and think it might require more help. This is a heavier, thicker arrangement that may hydrate looks that are too dry. While night creams are meant to provide your skin an extra dose of moisture while you sleep, day creams may be used as a foundation for makeup. Apply before causing a stir in the community, and you'll be greeted with soft, beautiful skin in the morning.

Oils: Consider oils if you really want to become even more saturated. Some oils may be a fantastic option for those with normal, sensitive, or dry skin. However, you should avoid using oil-saturating products if you have a tendency to break out easily or struggle with the need for specially designed smooth skin cosmetics.

Half the battle is figuring out how to apply cream correctly. Transfer a little amount onto your fingertips; the contact should ideally be around the size of a quarter. Start by applying the cream to your brow, working your way up and outward from the center of your face. At that time, apply the cream all over your cheeks in a similar manner, starting at your nose. Make sure you've applied the cream evenly across your skin in an effort to avoid clogging your pores. Once you've covered it enough with lotion, gently massage in circles, and wait a few minutes for it to dry before going on to the next step.

Stage 2: Establishing the Scene: The woman applies base makeup on her face.

Now that your skin is well hydrated, prepare your face with a primer. Groundwork is an important first step, whether of whether you want to apply a complete face of makeup or just a light coating of establishment. Applying primer underneath your makeup can prolong the appearance of your makeup.

What exactly is groundwork, then? Think about prepping a foundation for your makeup or cosmetics to help them apply more smoothly and stay longer. Groundworks are opulent gels and creams that optimize the material for your makeup by smoothing uneven surfaces and filling in all of the creases and pores.

Apply your introduction very lightly with your fingers or your preferred makeup brush or wipe. Master Tip: A little quantity has a big impact. Start with a dime-sized amount of primer in the center of your face and work your way outward to your cheekbones, temple, and jaw.

Find a dedicated product for the area of your face around your eyelids to apply foundation to the sensitive skin there (and maintain that professionally applied smokey eye look all day). Over the course of the day, oil from our eyelids may accumulate, giving the appearance of "wrinkled" eyeshadow. If you apply eyeshadow or eyeliner without first priming and your eyelids are smooth, the result might be uneven and asymmetrical.

Step 3: Foundation
A woman applying a liquid foundation to her face as part of her makeup routine.
Finding the right skin tone for you is the most important thing to consider when choosing an institution. An establishment's choice of shade may make a big difference. How then would you go about choosing? Compare the establishment tones with the shape of your face. After applying, you've located your true match in the unlikely event that the

establishment disappears with almost no mingling. Gaining some leeway to choose the ideal hue may require some trial and error, but it is important.

Once you've selected an item, think about the tools you'll need to apply it. Some women like to use their fingers, while others choose to use quality tools like brushes and wipes. If you're looking for a subtle highlight, your fingers might be the perfect tool. However, always wash them after applying makeup and avoid touching your face without fully cleaning them first. You don't want your fingerprints all over the place. Use an elegance blender or tool brush for an even more comprehensive effect.

Start in the center of your face and blend the liquid foundation outward. Don't forget to buff it in as you clear your establishment over the skin. Some women prefer to apply a damp cloth to their establishment to help ensure that it reaches the creases and wrinkles, resulting in a more equal and smoother surface. Additionally, some types of makeup brushes are ideal for blending in with the skin.

Step 4: Concealer

Woman applying concealer dots under her eyes as part of her beauty regimen

Concealer falls into two primary categories: stick/compact and liquid.

When you want to cover a significant portion of your face with light coverage, liquid concealer works well. If you want to achieve a dewy look, liquid concealer is also a great option, especially for crow's feet and mouth creases.

Concealers that are stick or compact work well for applying additional coverage to smaller, more focused regions of the face.

Choosing Your Concealer's Color

Purchasing two tones of concealer is a smart move. One that can be used to cover up pimples, dark spots, and other facial imperfections should be extremely similar to your skin tone. The other, which ought to be paler than your skin tone, can be utilized to draw attention to specific facial features or provide definition to your makeup style.

Note: Concealer is applied first by some ladies, then liquid foundation. It really is up to personal preference and trial and error which order to do these two stages in. Try both and see which technique gives your skin the smoothest, most luminous finish. Both are available in the Colorescience Finishing Touch Protocol product line, along with everything else you need to finish your look! On the other hand, you should always use concealer before powder foundation.

Where to Use a Concealer

Apply light concealer under the eyes using a moist sponge or makeup brush to minimize the appearance of dark under-eye circles and to produce a bright, radiant look. You may also want to use a dark circle cream.

Apply concealer precisely to the areas that need it to decrease the appearance of flaws.

Using a liquid or cream concealer, highlight the following parts of your face with tiny dots:

across the middle of your forehead horizontally
down the middle of your nose
beneath your gaze
Just behind your bottom lip, in a curved arch at the top of your chin
Cover it with a foundation or setting powder and gently blend it into the surrounding skin.

Step Five: FOUNDATION POWDER

Woman using her cosmetics brush to apply foundation powder
Applying foundation powder may be difficult; if you use too much, you'll have the dreaded "cake look," and if you use too little, you might as well have

skipped the step entirely. You've probably heard a lot of tips and techniques about powder foundation in your search for the perfect complexion. Remember these suggestions to achieve the ideal complexion.

Start by applying a thin layer of powder to your entire face using a big, fluffy powder brush. Using long, flowing strokes, press the bristles into the powder and then comb across the skin.

Applying a little extra powder could be helpful if you have certain regions of your skin that require additional coverage (the center of your face is usually where the red and greasy areas are). This step helps the powder enter pores and lines for a smoother texture by dipping your brush into the powder and pressing it firmly into the skin.

You won't even realize you're wearing makeup! The mineral powder product from Colorescience is lightweight, simple to use, and maintains the brightness and vibrancy of your skin.

Step Six: BRONZER

Woman holding up her portable mirror and applying bronzer cosmetics to her face

You may achieve a year-round sun-kissed shine on your complexion by using bronzer. To achieve a golden tan on your face, use a specialized bronzer brush. These brushes have more bristles and are packed much closer together, so you can get the most out of your vibrant bronzer with every swipe.

How to Pick the Correct Bronzer Shade

Selecting the incorrect bronzer shade is one of the most frequent mistakes people make. Use a bronzer that is no more than two shades darker than your skin tone if you're not experienced using one.

Where to Use Bronzer

Once you've chosen the appropriate shade, use your bronzer to create the number "3" on both cheeks.

Beginning at your forehead, drag the bronzer down your cheekbones and finally run it down your jawline, all the way to your chin. Expert Advice: Remember to integrate it with your neck. On the other side, repeat.

Step 7: BLUSH

A woman applying blush to her cheekbones. For decades, plumped cheekbones have been a staple of glamorous makeup. Blush could be the solution if you want to give your complexion a little more color and brightness. To ensure you get the most out of each blush sweep, apply your blush with a brush that is dense and has many of bristles.

Where to Use Blush

When it comes to blush application, there is no one-size-fits-all solution. To assist you select where to apply your blush, consider its hue.

Pink blush: Only apply pink blush to the apples of your cheeks when using it. The purpose of pink blush is to imitate the flush that naturally occurs in your body when blood gathers in your cheeks. Put on your finest smile to find the apples of your cheeks. The front portion of the cheek that accentuates when you smile is referred to as the "apple."

Plum blush: Similar to how light pink blush is used by people with fair complexions, plum blush can be applied by those with medium to dark skin tones.

Peach blush: Use these tones to assist shape your face and offer a subtle pop of color, as opposed to applying pink blush only to the apples of your cheeks. Turn one side of your face around (as if you were putting your lips together and pointing them in the other direction). Next, apply a peach blush to your cheekbones, tracing a line from your ears to the apples of your cheeks.

Step 8: Highlighter

On a table are highlighter cosmetics and a makeup brush.

Every makeup look is enhanced with a dash of glamour and shine by the appropriate highlighter. Highlighter may be used in addition to makeup, whether you're going for a more natural appearance or something dramatic and gorgeous.

Highlighters come in a variety of forms, including as liquids, creams, and powders. You may choose to use one, or find your favorite combination of many. Whatever option you choose, the application cycle carries on as before.

Where to Use a Highlighter

Once you've created a flawless timetable for your new firm, outline the whole area you want to highlight.

First, using a liquid highlighter, apply in the following areas:

Along the nose scaffolding
all the way over the tops of your cheekbones

inside the corners of your closed eyes
on the bone of your temple
The depression over your top lip, often known as the
Cupid's Bow
The center of attention in your temple
The main feature of your jawline
Once you're satisfied with the way your liquid
highlighter looks, blend it in with your fingers or a
wipe. Apply a coat of cream or powder highlighter
over the areas you want to draw attention to in order
to enhance the effect of your features.

all the way over the tops of your cheekbones
inside the corners of your closed eyes
on the bone of your temple
The depression over your top lip, often known as the
Cupid's Bow
The center of attention in your temple
The main feature of your jawline
Once you're satisfied with the way your liquid
highlighter looks, blend it in with your fingers or a
wipe. Apply a coat of cream or powder highlighter

over the areas you want to draw attention to in order to increase the effect of your featuring.

Boost your appearance and present your best self! Colorescience provides everything you need to achieve healthy, beautiful skin.

Step 9: EYESHADOW

Woman using makeup on her eyelids as part of her daily beauty routine.
Whether you choose muted hues or go bold with vivid tints, eyeshadow can liven up your makeup appearance. Select two matching eyeshadow shades for each appearance you choose: a lighter shade and a hazier shade.

After dipping your eyeshadow brush into the light shade, tap it to remove any excess pigment. Starting at the lash line and ending just above the folds on your eyelid, apply the lighter shadow over the whole upper lid.

Now, plunge your brush into the hazier variety once again, tapping off the excess. Simply apply the variation over your lash line in the outer corner of your eye. Remove the hazier kind from beneath your forehead bone and across your eyelid wrinkles. Applying makeup toward your eyelid's center should be stopped as you don't want to cover up the inner corners. Combine the two hues with a high-quality shadow brush. Apply the hazier shadow once more if you'd like a more somber appearance.

Step Ten: Eyeliner
Woman carefully lining her eyes with eyeliner

Applying eyeliner may be difficult; one mistake can result in "raccoon" eyes, which are not to be taken lightly. Use these basic eyeliner application techniques to overcome your makeup mishaps.

Types of Eyeliner

Fluid eyeliner: Your new best friend, if precision is what you're after, is fluid eyeliner. Fluid liners, which are applied with a fine plunging brush, are found in bottle structures. Moreover, fluid liner is available in marker-style pens.

Application instructions: Start thinly at the inner corner of your eye with fluid eyeliner, then gradually build up to the outside corner. Start drawing in the inner corner or the middle of your eye, and try to keep the tip of your liner or brush as close to your lash line as possible. Make tiny runs down the lash line with your liner brush by using tiny strokes, and then connect them to fill in any gaps. In the unlikely event that your hand slips, you can unwind! Clean up the area with a Q-tip dampened with a little amount of eye makeup remover.

Gel liner: Usually, this kind of liner comes in a little container with a tiny brush for application. For creating a feline eye appearance, gel eyeliner is fantastic.

The best technique to use is: A level, rakish brush should be dipped into the gel eyeliner pot. Make

sure both sides of the brush have the product on them by twirling it, then start applying from the lash line and go outward. Next, draw a line that divides the two lines, extending from the inner corner of your eye to the middle.
The finest eyeliner option for beginners is usually pencil eyeliner. Applying a pencil eyeliner with a pointed tip is an easy way to create a smokey eye on your waterline.

The best technique to employ is to sharpen your liner pencil after each usage. Draw tiny little specks starting at the outside corner of your upper eyelid after yanking your eyelid tight. To create a delicate dabbed line as close to the lash line as possible, work your way toward the inner corner of your eye. Use your pencil to sketch a clear conclusion, or use a small shadow brush to blend them in.

Step Eleven: MASCARA
Woman looking in the mirror as she applies mascara to her eyelashes

In the unlikely event that you will use only one makeup item, mascara should be the first thing on your list. Your eyes may seem more gorgeous with only a few mascara swipes in one easy action.

Many types of mascara are available, however the most well-known are usually the black and brown ones. Start by using an eyelash styler to twist your lashes.

The best technique for twisting your eyelashes is:

Making sure not to snag any of the sensitive skin around your eyelid, place the styler at the base of your top lashes.
Slowly shut off the styler.
Keep it configured for a few seconds.
Release gently
Once your lashes are twisted, grab your mascara container. Gently rotate the wand to ensure that all of the fibers are coated with mascara. Expert Tip: To avoid your mascara bunching, avoid squeezing the wand inside the cylinder as this allows air to enter.

Carefully stroke the mascara brush over your lashes' underlying roots. As a result, your lashes will have extra volume that you may apply to the tips. Get a clean wand and brush through your lashes if they are bunching together. For more volume, apply a second layer.

Step 12: Lip Glitter

The woman making lip gloss popular during her makeup routine

Prepare your lips before applying Gleam. If your lips are cracked and dry, be sure to use a gentle lip cleanser to remove any dead skin and a protective lip gloss. Next, use a lip balm or conditioner to help plump up your lips. Smear any excess once your lip salve has held its shape.

Beginning at the center of your lips, apply your lip glitter by dragging the tool the whole length of your furrowed brow. Try not to drag any glitter over your natural lip line, and gently lick your lips together to ensure that your lip gloss reaches all of your lips' tiny hiding places.

Step 13: Setting spray and powder.
The last step in your makeup routine might be setting powder and setting spray. Investing in a high-quality setting solution is crucial if you require makeup to last the whole day without lubricating, creasing, or glinting.

All skin types may benefit from setting showers, which can be used to establish various looks, such as wearing a full face of gorgeous makeup or just a little addition. Organizing your spray helps you minimize the need for reapplication of makeup and maintains the flawless appearance of your cosmetics for extended periods of time.

Setting spray are used in much the same way as applying hairspray to your jazzy do, and they provide the similar purpose for your face. Hold the bottle about eight inches away from your face. Then, lightly mist your face a few times to make sure every area is coated. Should you like to ensure that your makeup covers everything from your brow to your jawline, spray your face in an X form first, and then a T shape.

Once applied, there's a strong need to concentrate on the splash since it will dry quickly.

Final thought

Your makeup is complete. Whether you're heading straight to the office or going out for a memorable evening, it's easy to create a variety of outstanding appearances with these techniques for applying makeup.

Using Your Discretion to Raise the Bar for Your Cosmetics

Alright, now that we've covered the essentials and provided you with a foundation for a step-by-step cosmetics application method, we need to share with you a few more ideas that ought to become apparent when you make optional choices to elevate your cosmetics emphasis. What specifically would we have in care, all in all? Go on reading to learn more.

False Eyelashes

Not everyone has the privilege of being a member of the thick, lengthy, and twisted lash club. For that reason, if this seems true to you, don't sweat it. Fake eyelashes may be applied easily and are capable of deeper exploration. You may apply them skillfully at a lash salon or shop, or you can connect them yourself using a lash stick.

They may stay on for hours to weeks, depending on the lashes you choose and how you apply them! Therefore, depending on the method you choose, this step may be integrated in near the mascara application stage or it can completely replace that step. Having long, thick lashes may help draw attention to and enhance the appearance of your eyes.

CLEAN UP YOUR BRUSHES

You may think that this optional step won't have a greater impact, but when your brushes are clean, everything is working to give your makeup the greatest chance of applying evenly and powerfully. Additionally, you can rest easy knowing that you have discovered a genuine method to ensure that your materials and cosmetics are as free of tiny organisms as possible. We promise that your skin will appreciate it later.

ADDITIONAL ITEMS FOR YOUR TRUCK

When your basic supply of makeup is nearly depleted, you should make sure you replenish it and buy the items you are running low on before they really run out. In the unlikely event that you wait too long, you may find yourself unable to create the desired appearance. That is also uncomfortable for everyone.

Chapter 6: Staying Ahead of Beauty Trends

To remain on top of things for magnificence drifts, it's fundamental to effectively search out data and teach yourself on what's coming straightaway. Follow forces to be reckoned with and magnificence organizations.

• Tips on staying ahead of beauty trends

Follow your #1 effects via online entertainment:
This is one of the least demanding ways of keeping awake to date on magnificence trends.You can follow hashtags that connect with beauty,like #beautytrends. You can evaluate new things from them like hair,outfits, cosmetics looks or anything that interest you

Peruse excellence magazines: This is one more method for getting in top of magnificence patterns from understanding magazines .like vogue,allure and others
Watch magnificence recordings eg youtube:

You can get incredible assets from excellence videos,and you can find out about new items from watching recordings from magnificence forces to be reckoned with.

Go to excellence occasion:

You can think about going to excellence occasions. This are incredible approaches to meeting other magnificence aficionados.

Shop from puts that are on top on excellence pattern: When you shop from shops that are on top on magnificence patterns, you make certain to get the most recent forward-thinking magnificence item.

The most effective method to remain sound cognizant while keeping steady over patterns

● Tips to stay healthy conscious while staying on tip of trends

Do your research: Before attempting another item or pattern generally do all necessary investigation on that item prior to utilizing it, read surveys and counsel a wellbeing proficient.

Stick to regular items: Consistently stick to normal items, keep away from items created with synthetics.

Be careful of recent fads: Few out of every odd pattern is worth trying,some can be extremely hazardous. So be very cautious,some sounds unrealistic.

Try not to feel like you should keep with each pattern: Figure out how to pick the one that you feel alright with.

Consider your skin type: Not all patterns are reasonable for all skin types. Continuously consider your skin while picking excellence items. Assuming you are slick skin keep away from item that are oily in nature,if you are dry skin keep away from items that have drying properties.

Pay attention to your body: In the event that you begin utilizing an item and you begin having response, kindly stop it.

Chapter 7: Expert Beauty Advice

With regards to our skin or our face we search for the best excellence tips and in the event that these come from proficient magnificence specialists, these excellence tips are what we as a whole search for. Magnificence privileged insights for shining, faultless, or perhaps sound skin is certainly not a one day approach, it must be a standard system with some additional consideration. Proficient excellence specialists sharing their magnificence insider facts can be the best excellence tips for us.

Why Excellence Tips from Proficient Magnificence Specialists As it were?

An expert stunner expert is a specialist in magnificence, skin and body care items. They prompt their clients on the best items and the correct method for minding subsequent to breaking down the kind of skin according to the particular necessities. Accordingly when you want the most recent and best excellence tips for your skin and body you ought to constantly pay attention to master guidance.

- **Insights from skincare and beauty experts**

1. Utilize the right product for your skin type.
"For sleek or skin break out inclined skin, a salicylic gel or benzoyl peroxide wash

works perfectly. For dry mature skin, utilize either a saturating glycolic or smooth cleaning agent. For skin with earthy colored spots or melasma, utilize a lighting up wash, like an alpha hydroxy corrosive chemical."

2. Try not to utilize an excessive number of items.

Layering on numerous skincare items at the same time is a major no, It tends to be unforgiving on the skin, bringing about additional breakouts and obstructed pores.

3. Saturate both constantly.

"The best times to saturate are just after you escape the shower and just before you head to sleep," Keep away from creams with weighty scents and ensure you find a lotion delicate enough for each day use with zero bothering.

4. Try not to contact your face.

Try work on some way to try not to contact your face is vital. It doesn't simply spread microorganisms and cause breakouts — it can prompt scarring, an expansion in kinks, and, surprisingly, influenza or other infections.

5. Hydrate all around.

Each skin master we addressed accentuated the significance of hydration. "An absence of water implies not so much brilliance but rather more list," says Dr. Mona Gohara, a dermatologist in Connecticut. She proposes picking items (purging, saturating, and against maturing) that have hydrating recipes. Furthermore, obviously, drink around eight glasses of water a day.

6. Stay away from direct intensity openness.

Try not to simply keep an eye out for the sun — getting excessively near radiators and chimneys can likewise unleash devastation on your skin. "It causes aggravation and collagen breakdown. I suggest remaining somewhere around ten feet away," makes sense of Dr. Debbie Palmer, a New York dermatologist. So whenever you're simmering chestnuts or s'mores over an open fire, make a stride back.

7. Two or multiple times for every week.

"We lose 50 million skin cells daily, and without some additional bump, they might stick around leaving the skin looking dismal. To battle this, you ought to "pick an item that is pH impartial so it doesn't dry as it sheds." And don't stop with your face — the skin on your body needs peeling, as well.

8. Nutrients ought to go on your skin, as well.

A fair eating regimen is significant, yet there's more than one method for giving your skin nutrients. There are likewise skin cancer prevention agents, which are serums and creams that contain fixings that support the skin (think L-ascorbic acid serum!).

"These can truly assist with fixing the skin from sun harm. Not certain how to utilize them? The best opportunity to apply them is just subsequent to purging so your skin can absorb them, or they can be layered under your sunscreen for added assurance.

9. Get your greens.

However it's enticing to snatch an espresso the moment you awaken, Joanna Vargas, a skincare facialist in New York City, says picking the right refreshments can be a distinct advantage. "Drink an injection of chlorophyll each day to light up, oxygenate, and hydrate your skin. Drinking chlorophyll likewise helps channel puffiness by invigorating the lymphatic framework, so it's additionally great for cellulite."

In the event that you're not enthused about bringing down a dose of the stuff, chlorophyll enhancements can be found at numerous pharmacies and wellbeing food stores. She likewise educated drinking green juices with parcels concerning veggies in them: "It will change your skin surprisingly fast — and it oxygenates the skin and animates lymphatic seepage, so it's de-puffing, as well."

10. Keep a solid eating regimen.

"Your skin has a characteristic boundary to hold dampness, and vital for that is omega-3 unsaturated fat. "Flax seeds on your plate of mixed greens or even pecans will be a moment lift to your omega-3, in this manner expanding your skin's capacity to clutch dampness." And make certain to eat an eating routine low in food sources with a high glycemic file (straightforward and complex carbs).

11. Clean your cosmetics brushes routinely.

To battle disease and stopped up pores, wash concealer and establishment brushes one time per week. For brushes you use around your eyes, she suggests two times a month, and for some other brushes, when a month is fine.

This is how it's done: Put a drop of a gentle cleanser into the center of your hand. Wet the fibers with tepid water. Then, knead the fibers into your palm to disseminate the cleanser into the brush. Try not to get the metal piece of the brush wet/or the foundation of the brush hairs in light of the fact that the paste could mellow and the fibers could drop out. Flush the cleanser out and press out the water with a towel. Lay the brushes on their side with the fibers draping off the edge of the counter to dry.

12. Wear sunscreen 365 days every year. Regardless, inside or out.

"Many individuals feel they possibly need to safeguard themselves on radiant days or while visiting the ocean side. "Yet, truly we want to safeguard our skin in any event, while we're driving a vehicle, flying in a plane, or getting things done. The everyday UV openness adds to the apparent indications of maturing." What sort of sunscreen is ideal? Pick a wide range sunscreen with a SPF of 30 or more prominent — and recollect that it should be reapplied like clockwork.

13. Sun insurance doesn't stop at sunscreen.

We're talking SPF cosmetics, shades, and expansive overflowed caps. "Forestalling sun harm is multiple times preferred for your skin over treating it sometime later," says Dr. Prystowsky.

14. Work on your skincare schedule.

"Craze items and extravagant fixings are enjoyable to attempt, and once in a while they function admirably," says Dr. Prystowsky, "however generally they're off the racks similarly as fast as they're on them." Track down a cleaning agent and lotion that you know work for you, and keep them at the center of your daily practice.

15. Rest more brilliant.

It's not just about getting eight hours every evening. Skin will likewise profit from routinely utilizing clean silk pillowcases. "The material skims effectively and forestalls wrinkling and wrinkles"Silk is additionally more straightforward on hair

— it maintains a strategic distance from tangles and breakage." Better hair and skin while you rest? Certainly.

Chapter 8: Beauty Secrets Unveiled

Magnificence insider facts, those prized tips and deceives gave over through ag2es have forever been, at the cutting edge of the excellence business. They include an assortment of monitored procedures that assist people with taking advantage of their excellence potential. From skincare customs to cosmetics hacks these mysteries hold importance in the realm of excellence.

The magnificence business is truly developing contribution a scope of items and techniques to improve one's appearance. Anyway the protected magnificence mysteries frequently have the sorcery to change your search in manners others can hardly comprehend. They award admittance to procedures utilized by industry specialists opening ways to brilliance and certainty.

By integrating these excellence mysteries into your normal you can improve your general appearance in noteworthy ways. Powerful skincare tips guarantee a radiant tone while cosmetics stunts emphasize your elements easily featuring your regular magnificence. These privileged insights enable people to embrace their properties and express their beauty and appeal.

• **Expert tips for ageless beauty**

A. The Meaning of Predictable Skincare Schedule

Keeping a reliable skincare routine is pivotal, for keeping your skin sound and brilliant. By following a routine you can successfully scrub, saturate and safeguard your skin from harm. Consistency assumes a part, in accomplishing results.

B. Ways to keep your skin solid and brilliant

Ensure you drink a lot of water over the course of the day to keep your skin appropriately hydrated.

To safeguard your skin from the UV beams of the sun apply sunscreen on a premise.

Purify your face a day to kill soil, oil and pollutants.

Routinely shed to dispose of skin cells and advance the turnover of cells.

Keep your skin saturated to keep up with its hydration and flexibility.

C. Privileged insights for tending to skincare concerns

1. Managing skin inflammation skin

Assuming you have skin inflammation skin it's vital to utilize delicate, non comedogenic and oil free items. Keep away from chemicals. Pick fixings like salicylic corrosive or benzoyl peroxide that actually target skin inflammation causing microbes.

2. Fighting dried out skin

To battle got dried out skin integrate a hydrating serum or lotion into your skincare schedule. Search for fixings like corrosive, glycerin and ceramides that renew dampness levels and reestablish your skins obstruction.

3. Tending to maturing signs on the skin

To handle indications of maturing like lines and kinks pick items that contain cell reinforcements, similar to L-ascorbic acid or retinol.
These fixings can possibly upgrade the versatility of your skin, support collagen creation and slowly diminish the presence of kinks.

• Inside beauty hacks

Opening the Key to Immaculate Skin

Cosmetics has the capacity to highlight your excellence and totally change your appearance. By utilizing methods and using quality items you can achieve a cosmetics base and make hypnotizing cosmetics looks. Here are some restrictive excellence hacks that will lift your magnificence game:

A. Methods, for accomplishing a perfect cosmetics base

Start by setting up your skin with a lotion and preliminary which will lay out a material for putting on cosmetics.

Use tone amending concealer to kill any defects like redness or dark circles.

Apply establishment utilizing a cosmetics wipe for a characteristic completion.

Set your establishment with powder to draw out its life span.

B. Bit by bit instructional exercises for cosmetics looks

Figure out how to easily accomplish a cosmetics look.

Disclose the privileged insights behind making a smokey eye for night occasions.

Excel at creating dynamic cosmetics looks appropriate for events.

C. Tips, for enduring cosmetics application

Use a setting shower to guarantee that your cosmetics stays set up over the course of the day without smirching or dissolving endlessly.

Pick enduring and waterproof items for your eyeliner, mascara and lipstick to guarantee they wait over the course of the day.

Make sure to smear any oil from your face during the day to keep a looking cosmetics application.

● Secret to a healthy lifestyle and nutrition for beauty

Keep a fair eating regimen for sound skin and hair by remembering different foods grown from the ground for your feasts that give fundamental nutrients and cell reinforcements.
Support hair. Strength by consolidating proteins, similar to fish, chicken or beans into your eating regimen.

Pick sugars such, as grains to keep your energy levels consistent and support the strength of your skin. It's ideal to try not to eat measures of handled food sources as they can prompt skin aggravation and breakouts.

Presently lets discuss how you can integrate food sources that upgrade magnificence into your feasts. Incorporate food sources that're wealthy in omega 3 acids like salmon and pecans as they sustain the skin and give it a sound shine. You can likewise add berries and dull chocolate to your eating regimen as they are high in cell reinforcements that safeguard the skin from harm brought about by revolutionaries. Remember to incorporate carrots and citrus natural products for nutrients An and C which assist with collagen creation and keeping up with skin flexibility. Finally integrating zinc rich food sources like clams and pumpkin seeds can advance hair development while forestalling balding.

Hydration is urgent for keeping a coloring and an energetic appearance. Ensure you hydrate consistently in light of the fact that it helps hydrate the skin diminishing the perceivability of lines and kinks. Furthermore remaining hydrated helps flush out poisons from your body prompting skin, with flaws. It likewise works on the versatility and flexibility of your skin while advancing a scalp that limits hair dryness and breakage.

Ensure you drink at eight glasses of water consistently to keep your skin and hair hydrated and looking their very best.

Normal activity is indispensable, for upgrading excellence as it further develops wellbeing while at the same time helping blood course. This expanded blood stream conveys supplements and oxygen to the skin cells bringing about a coloring. Practice likewise decreases feelings of anxiety. Advances rest, prompting a revived appearance. Besides, remaining dynamic improves pose which thusly gives you an energetic position.

To target region of the body as per your excellence objectives integrating practices that attention on those areas is pivotal.

To accomplish an etched figure it's critical to incorporate strength preparing practices in your daily schedule. Center around developments, similar to squats, thrusts and deadlifts to focus on your glutes, thighs and center muscles. To upgrade consuming and by and large muscle definition matching these activities with cardiovascular exercises like running or cycling is suggested.

Assuming that you're searching for a characterized waistline, focus on practices that connect with your muscles. Consider integrating side boards and Russian turns into your gym routine everyday practice.

To foster versatile arms it's gainful to incorporate activities, for example, push ups, rear arm muscle plunges and bicep twists. These developments will assist with conditioning your arms while developing fortitude in the muscle gatherings.

For a firm bum integrating practices like glute spans, hip pushes and jackass kicks into your routine can. Shape your glutes really.

To accomplish a thin and conditioned back while further developing stance have a go at including works out, similar to lat pull downs, twisted around lines and Superman presents. These developments will reinforce the muscles in your back.

Presently lets investigate a few privileged insights that can assist you with keeping a wellness schedule

Put forth objectives: Begin with goals that line up with your ongoing wellness level. Steadily increment the power and span of your exercises as you progress.

Track down exercises: Pick practices that you really appreciate doing so they become a piece of your daily schedule.
Whether its moving, swimming or going on climbs enjoying exercises can add to keeping a daily schedule.

Remain coordinated: Plan your activity meetings somewhat early. Integrate them into your timetable. Treat your exercise time as a responsibility, to yourself.

Track down an exercise mate: Get a companion or relative to go along with you on your wellness process. Practicing together can make it more charming. Give the inspiration and backing.

Reward yourself: Commend the achievements and accomplishments you arrive at en route. Indulge yourself with a day at the spa. Enjoy a sound prize as a wellspring of proceeded with inspiration.

Chapter 9: Beauty Hacks for Busy Lives

In the present quick moving world, carving out opportunity for taking care of oneself, not to skincare routine can challenge. However, dealing with your skin is fundamental for keeping up with solid, gleaming, and brilliant skin. Fortunately, with a couple of skincare hacks, you can keep your skin sound without forfeiting an excess of time. Here are some skincare hacks for occupied individuals.

Keep it straightforward

Twofold purify
Use performing multiple tasks items
Saturate in a hurry
Remember your neck and hands
Use sheet covers

Remain hydrated

With regards to skincare, toning it down would be ideal. You needn't bother with a ten-step routine to keep your skin solid. As a matter of fact, utilizing such a large number of items can hurt your skin, prompting disturbance, breakouts, and dryness. All things considered, center around involving a couple of fundamental items that work for your skin type. A straightforward everyday practice of purifying, saturating, and sun security can do some incredible things for your skin.

Twofold purge

Twofold purging is a distinct advantage with regards to skincare. It includes utilizing an

oil-based chemical to eliminate cosmetics and soil, trailed by a water-based cleaning agent to clean the skin. Twofold purifying guarantees that all hints of soil, oil, and cosmetics are taken out from the skin, leaving it perfect and revived.
Use performing various tasks items
Performing various tasks items are a gift from heaven for occupied individuals. Search for items that can fill different needs, for example, a colored lotion with SPF, a cream with cell reinforcements, or a serum with hyaluronic corrosive and L-ascorbic acid. These items can set aside you time and cash while as yet furnishing your skin with the vital supplements.

Cream in a hurry
In the event that you're generally in a hurry, you might have the opportunity to apply lotion in the first part of the day. Notwithstanding, keeping a lotion in your sack can assist you with saturating over the course of the day. Search for a

lightweight cream that the skin can without much of a stretch retain, like a gel or a serum. Serum serum is a phenomenal choice for saturating in a hurry. Loaded with hyaluronic corrosive and miniature squalene containers, it's your definitive hydration station. On the off chance that you're a cosmetics wearer, pick a saturating spritz you can top up over your cosmetics.

Remember your neck and hands

Your neck and hands are many times disregarded with regards to skincare. Nonetheless, they are many times the main regions to give indications of maturing. Try to stretch out your skincare routine to your neck and hands by utilizing similar items you use all over.

Use sheet covers

Sheet covers are a speedy and simple method for providing your skin with an increase in hydration and supplements. They can be utilized while you're doing different things, like staring at the television or chipping away at your PC. Search for sheet veils that focus on your particular skin concerns, like dryness, bluntness, or skin inflammation. FOREO has a variety of Ranch to Face sheet veils for each need. Green tea to stimulate and light up the skin, Coconut Oil to sustain the skin, and Acai berry for an increase in cell reinforcements FOREO has everything.

Remain hydrated

Drinking sufficient water is fundamental for keeping your skin hydrated and solid. Plan to drink something like eight glasses of water everyday to keep your skin brilliant.

Dealing with your skin doesn't need to be tedious or muddled. By following these skincare hacks, you can keep your skin sound and sparkling, regardless of whether you have a bustling timetable. Keep in mind, the key is to keep it basic, use performing multiple tasks items and remain hydrated.

- ## Time saving tricks for a busy lifestyle

It's essential to deal with a bustling timetable to expand effectiveness and efficiency. Executing compelling using time effectively and booking strategies can assist you with streamlining your typical business day for most extreme execution. Dealing with a bustling timetable can show current and future managers your capacity to sort out your endeavors, self-regulate your errands and complete both complicated and straightforward obligations in an opportune and excellent manner.

Here are procedures you can use to arrange your bustling timetable:

1. Partition huge errands into more modest ones

In the event that a task could require hours, days, weeks or longer to finish, you can take a stab at sharing the venture's means. Doing this can assist you with partaking in a progression of little achievements and gradually pursue the essential objective. You can likewise abstain from feeling overpowered by following through with a perplexing job in more modest, less complex advances. For instance, in the event that you want to set up a 50-page worker manual, you can separate the manual by parts and segments inside every section. As you complete each part, you progress toward the fruition of the entirety.

2. Focus on your work

Focusing on your work can assist you with finishing the most basic responsibilities first, which might assist with freeing sentiments from stress or vulnerability. There are numerous ways of focusing on errands, for example, by closest cutoff times, the significance of the client, individual significance to you and unique solicitations by the executives. By finishing these high-need errands first, you might find that you feel less strain in your typical business day on the grounds that the most pressing work is now finished.

3. Screen your time

Checking how much time it takes for you to get done with each job can help you all the more effectively grasp the region of your timetable that need consideration. You can keep a composed log or utilize a period following application to screen how long you spend doing various things.

When you know where you invest your energy everyday, you can ponder whether you really want to change any pieces of your daily practice. You can all the more rigorously control your time by setting cutoff times for your assignments. In some cases, having a cutoff time can urge you to rapidly follow through with your responsibilities more. You can set a clock to remind yourself to change to the following undertaking. Assuming you notice that you delay at specific times, consider setting your timetable to cover with the times you ordinarily are less useful to advance that time.

4. Plan your gatherings decisively

There are methodologies to diminish how much time you spend in gatherings while as yet guaranteeing that you accomplish your gathering objectives. You can consider whether the subject requires an in-person gathering or on the other hand on the off chance that you can orchestrate a virtual or telephone discussion to wipe out drive time.

Assuming a gathering is fundamental, you can lessen how much time that the gathering takes by sending the plan early, setting a relentless timetable, including end times, helping members to remember the excess time and keeping the quantity of individuals in participation moderately low. With less individuals, everybody can share their contribution to somewhat less time and you could find it simpler to keep the discussion on task.

5. Set reachable execution assumptions
In 1. Your capacities might shift relying upon the day, so it's critical to invest a touch of energy every morning really pondering how much things you can sensibly hope to finish.

6. Delegate or rethink a portion of your errands

Now and again, you can find someone else who can do part or all of a portion of your errands to assist you with zeroing in on different obligations. Contingent upon your situation, you might have the option to recognize who can take on a portion of your obligations and relegate the errands to them.

You can likewise pay an external individual to finish a portion of your errands to let loose your functioning time. One model would employ a right hand to deal with your timetable and browse your messages, as well as ready you to the pressing ones and answer others.

7. Acknowledge how much work you can sensibly deal with

You might feel strain to acknowledge more work than you can practically finish. This could occur to dazzle directors in another position or on the other hand in the event that you're being considered for an advancement. Taking on more work than you can reasonably finish can at times prompt a decline in generally execution, like missed cutoff times and diminished work quality.

To stay away from this, you can allude to your timetable and look at whether as another undertaking is one that you can deal with to your norms. In the event that you don't feel you can finish the responsibility, speak the truth about your reasons while deferentially declining. Being particular about the positions you take on can assist with guaranteeing you can fulfill all of your time constraints and follow through on your commitments.

8. Keep a focal timetable

You could find it supportive to set up a solitary timetable in which you keep all of your day to day, week by week, month to month and longer-term undertakings. By having all of your to-do things in a focal area, you could find it simpler to rapidly check what you want to finish and whether have the opportunity to take on extra undertakings. This timetable could be advanced or physical, contingent upon what you see as generally agreeable. You can additionally arrange the timetable by variety coding undertakings by earnestness, type or due date.

9. Bunch errands

You might work on your proficiency and complete your assignments quicker by getting done with related or comparative responsibilities simultaneously. Clustering together related work can build proficiency and efficiency since it very well might be simpler to trade between undertakings that require a similar kind of work. These can incorporate things like noting messages, illustrating addresses, reviewing tasks or making plans. For instance, you could save a period on the last Monday of each and every month to make the financial plan for all divisions you regulate.

10. Use inescapable personal time

During your day, you might experience times when there is no particular task to take care of while you trust that the following assignment will begin. For instance, you could drive on the train or have a 10-or 15-minute hole between a progression of gatherings. You could utilize that time by doing things like noting messages or perusing brief articles.

Consider setting up a rundown early on of more modest errands that you can finish during these times of spare energy. After some time, these minor undertakings can amount to a lot of useful time that you could some way or another not use proficiently.

11. Plan consistently

Certain individuals find it supportive to make a day to day timetable to ensure they have achieved immeasurably significant errands every day. You can make your following day's timetable toward the finish of your ongoing business day, around evening time before bed, in the first part of the day when you drink your espresso or any time that you feel generally prepared to ponder the following day's assignments.

At the point when you set up your timetable, there are a few techniques you can attempt to make the best utilization of your time. You can orchestrate your assignments to fit around the time you feel generally useful. For instance, certain individuals feel most stimulated in the first part of the day, some after lunch and some at night. You could organize your undertakings to finish troublesome or complex things first and perform assignments you appreciate more around the day's end. Or on the other hand, you can set the assignment that will require some investment for the start of the day.

12. Keep away from interruptions

While expanding the utilization of your time, it's critical to restrict and stay away from interruptions. You might find your work process hindered by a text or email notices or by representatives strolling into your office. In these examples, you can try not to be occupied from your ongoing errands and attempt to build your proficiency by putting your telephone on quiet, stopping your inbox, wearing earphones to show that you are occupied or shutting your office entryway.

13. Enjoy reprieves

Despite the fact that dawdling can be an issue on the off chance that it diminishes your proficiency and efficiency, booked breaks can be useful for some reasons. Assuming you plan for breaks and use them to unwind, eat, deal with individual assignments or contemplate things other than work, you could find that you have more energy and center when the time has come to work once more. The key is to plan these breaks and make them time-restricted to keep them from turning into a lingering device.

• Maintaining beauty on the go

1. Continue to apply lotion

Apply extraordinary saturating cream the prior night you travel. This will assist with keeping the skin hydrated and saturated and furthermore saves from the unfriendly weather patterns. Direct daylight or solid breeze can make the skin dry and harm the skin surface notably. Reapply the cream while going to keep a delicate, graceful skin, independent of the weather patterns.

2. Keep your skin hydrated

The lipid hindrance restrains dampness misfortune from the skin and shields it from natural aggressors. Apply a cream that reinforces the lipid boundary as well as keeps up with it as well. Go for a lotion that contains Fixings like hyaluronic corrosive, glycerin and L-ascorbic acid to support obstruction wellbeing.
Saturate your skin somewhere around two times day to day! Picture kindness: Shutterstock.

3. Continuously keep SPF helpful

Apply sunscreen liberally to save the skin from the cruel impacts of UV beams. It will assist with shielding the skin from tanning and sun related burns. Over the top openness to the sun additionally brings about early maturing.
Reapply it each 2-3 hourly and utilize a decent emollient to keep the skin soggy from the inside.
Burn from the sun side effects
Sun related burn might result from a lot of sun or delayed sun openness. Picture kindness: Shutterstock.

4. Apply a cleanser

While voyaging, our skin draws in a great deal of soil and residue which get gathered on the skin and cause breakouts. A cleanser will clean out all the grime and keep the skin spotless and revived. Keep your cleanser with you as even a slight change in skincare items might act unexpectedly on the skin and cause 'excursion breakouts'.

5. Apply toner

Keep a hydrating face fog convenient to quiet any redness or bothering on the skin. Keep a toner in your movement pocket as its plans can in a split second mattify and recharge sweat-soaked and oily skin. It likewise balances the pH levels of the skin so you experience the ill effects of no breakouts or bluntness later on.

Chapter 10: The Cosmetic industry

The restorative business depicts the business that makes and appropriates corrective items. These incorporate variety beauty care products, similar to establishment and mascara, skincare, for example, creams and chemicals, hair care, for example, shampoos, conditioners and hair tones, and toiletries, for example, bubble shower and cleanser. The assembling business is overwhelmed by few worldwide companies that started in the mid twentieth hundred years, yet the dissemination and offer of beauty care products is spread among an extensive variety of various businesses.Cosmetics should be protected when clients use them as per the name's directions or in the regular or anticipated way. One measure a maker might take to ensure the wellbeing of a restorative item is item trying. FDA once in a while does testing as a component of its examination program or while investigating potential security issues with an item. Both the beauty care products business and buyers can profit from the FDA's assets on item testing.

- ## **Exploring the world of beauty product**

Investigating the Universe of magnificence produces.Such as cosmetics, skincare items, aromas, and individual consideration things.

Beauty care products are fundamentally utilized for stylish purposes, assisting people with working on their appearance. This lifts their fearlessness or communicates their imagination through various looks and styles. They are accessible in different structures, including creams, salves, powders, gels, showers, and lipsticks, among others.

Self-Articulation and Innovativeness:

Beauty care products give a stage to self-articulation and innovativeness. They permit people to try different things with various varieties, styles, and looks, empowering them to communicate their extraordinary character, imaginative energy, or social impacts.

Expanded Fearlessness:

Utilizing beauty care products can emphatically affect confidence and self-assurance. At the point when people feel that they put their best self forward, it can help their certainty, work on their mental self portrait, and add to a good outlook.

Insurance and Sustenance:

Numerous restorative items, especially skincare items, offer defensive and supporting advantages for the skin and hair. Sunscreens safeguard against unsafe UV beams, lotions hydrate and sustain the skin, and hair care items assist with keeping up with solid and sensible hair.

Recognizing trustworthy brands and items

In all honesty, the FDA doesn't manage or characterize terms like "clean," "regular," "green," or even "natural" inside the magnificence business, permitting brands to guarantee their items as "clean excellence" with no genuine sponsorship or review. This cycle, characterized as greenwashing, is the point at which a brand deliberately deludes purchasers into accepting that their items are 100 percent protected and normal, while sneaking in poisonous (and possibly hurtful) fixings.

To exacerbate the situation, Phthalates, aggravations, and other known endocrine disruptors are totally legitimate in the US and are not expected to be revealed on fixing records or item bundling. The best way to guarantee item wellbeing and fixing virtue is to search for accreditation seals.

- **Identifying reputable brands and product**

1. Search for Unadulterated and Simple To-Track down Fixings

When in doubt of thumb, fixing records ought to be both simple to peruse and situate on a brand's site. On the off chance that the fixing list contains confounding terms that aren't made sense of, or on the other hand assuming that it takes many snaps to find the rundown on the site, it is conceivable the brand may be concealing something.

At Ogee, we unequivocally express the source from which every one of our recorded fixings are inferred to dispense with any disarray about logical phrasing. For instance, Hyaluronic Corrosive and Glycerin (from vegetable sources), Tocopherol (Vitamin E from Sunflower Oil), and Squalane (from Sugarcane).

Keep in mind, "scent" isn't a fixing and is a significant warning on any brand's fixing list. To make things considerably trickier, fixings are many times recorded under various names, so be on the chase after the poisonous fixings beneath!

We Never Formulate With:
artificial dye

X Manufactured Aromas

X Silicones

X Sulfates

X Parabens

X Petrochemicals

X Talc

X Hydroquinone

Our NSF Natural Certificate connotes that every item contains at least 70% natural substance and limits the leftover 30% to regular materials that were planned in a way that conforms to our natural qualities.

Since an item is "sans scent" doesn't mean it is spotless or natural. Our items contain normal, organically determined fragrances that are liberated from engineered synthetics, yet still give an unobtrusive and new smell.

We Really do Figure out With:

+ Regular Mineral Shades

+ Rose Concentrate

+ Alpha Hydroxy Acids (AHAs)

+ Frankincense Concentrate

+ Cold-Press Jojoba Oil

+ Natural Aloe Leaf Juice

+ Edelweiss Blossom Plant Undifferentiated cells

+ Sugarcane Determined Squalane

2. Search For Industry-Controlled Certificates

Search for seals from NSF, USDA, affirmed Non-GMO, Jumping Rabbit, Excellence Without Rabbits (PETA savagery free seal), and some other respectable affirmations.

At Ogee, our whole assortment has acquired Natural Certificate to the NSF Individual Consideration Standard to guarantee hands down the best and most secure fixings are utilized inside our plans.

3. Clear Standards and Brand Ethos

The most widely recognized way that brands "greenwash" customers is through their bundling and publicizing, so make certain to search for genuine seals and callouts on the brand's site and web-based entertainment accounts.

At Ogee, we put stock in full straightforwardness. We stick to natural and reasonable standards through our obligation to moral and fair strategic approaches with our providers, items, representatives, accomplices, and local area.

Ogee is 100 percent mercilessness free and maintains a severe no creature testing strategy under the Jumping Rabbit Confirmation. We encourage broad reception and improvement of natural cultivating frameworks through our glad help of the Natural Cultivating Exploration Establishment.

.

- ## **Making informed choice when shopping for cosmetics**

Presentation:
In the domain of skincare, the decisions are apparently perpetual, from serums and lotions to chemicals and toners.
With such countless choices accessible, one squeezing question emerges: Would it be a good idea for you to buy your skincare items from a drug store or a grocery store?

This article means to give you bits of knowledge and contemplations to assist you with pursuing an educated choice that lines up with your skincare needs and inclinations.

Grasping the Specific situation

Prior to plunging into the dynamic interaction, we should comprehend the particular qualities of buying skincare items from a drug store versus a grocery store.

Buying from a Drug store

Drug stores frequently convey an extensive variety of skincare items, a considerable lot of which are organized in view of dermatologist proposals. These foundations are exceptional to take care of explicit skin concerns and may offer better quality brands with demonstrated adequacy.

The presence of prepared drug specialists can be a significant resource, as they can offer customized counsel in light of your skin type and concerns.

Shopping at a General store

Grocery stores, then again, give accommodation and openness. They offer an assortment of skincare items that are by and large reasonable and simple to find.

While they might miss the mark on particular skill of drug specialists, stores can in any case offer notable brands and a choice of items reasonable for regular skincare schedules.

Variables to Consider

1. Skin Concerns

On the off chance that you're managing explicit skin concerns like skin inflammation, hyperpigmentation, or extreme responsiveness, buying from a drug store may be more useful. Drug specialists can offer customized counsel and suggest items supported by logical examination.

2. Ability

Drug stores give the benefit of having experts who figure out the subtleties of skincare fixings. They can direct you through fixing records and assist you with picking items that best suit your skin type and objectives.

3. Item Reach

Stores offer a more broad grouping of skincare items reasonable for regular use. In the event that you're searching for fundamental skincare things without explicit necessities, a grocery store may be a helpful decision.

4. Financial plan

While drug stores might offer very good quality brands with premium estimating, grocery stores will generally have a scope of reasonable choices. Consider your spending plan while going with a choice.

5. Comfort

General stores are normally more available and have longer working hours. In the event that you're searching for a speedy and basic skincare arrangement, general stores may be more reasonable.

Finally

Eventually, the choice between buying skincare items from a drug store or a grocery store reduces to your singular requirements and inclinations.

In the event that you're looking for master direction, particular items, and have explicit skin concerns, a drug store may be the better choice. Then again, in the event that you're searching for comfort and reasonableness without complex necessities, a grocery store could address your issues successfully.

Keep in mind, your skin merits the best consideration, so set aside some margin to explore items, read surveys, and talk with experts if vital.

By going with informed decisions, you're putting resources into your skin's wellbeing and your general prosperity.

Chapter 11:A Beauty Journey to Feel your best

Living in a general public that frequently extols a specific self-perception, it's not difficult to fall into the snare of self-analysis and disappointment with our own appearance. In any case, feeling better in your skin isn't subject to adjusting to cultural excellence norms. Genuine satisfaction and certainty come from inside as we figure out how to acknowledge and value our bodies, regardless of their shape or size. This week, we dig into the craft of embracing your body and give viable tips on developing self esteem and feeling content with yourself.

Acknowledgment is the key

The excursion to feeling better in your skin starts with self-acknowledgment. Recognize that everyone is special and lovely in their own particular manner. Contrasting yourself with others just encourages weakness. All things being equal, center around your assets and praise the characteristics that make you unique.

Carefully Taking care of oneself

Dealing with your body is a fundamental piece of feeling better in your skin. Practice taking care of oneself carefully, with next to no judgment or culpability. Sustain your body with nutritious food sources, remain hydrated, and participate in proactive tasks that give you pleasure. Keep in mind, taking care of oneself is tied in with treating yourself with generosity, not rebuffing yourself for not squeezing into erratic excellence norms.

DRESS FOR YOURSELF

Wear garments that cause you to feel good and certain. Style go back and forth, yet your style ought to mirror your character and inclinations. Embrace furnishes that fulfill you, no matter what's thought of "in" right now.

ENCIRCLE YOURSELF WITH ENERGY

Individuals we encircle ourselves with can fundamentally impact our self-insight. Search out companions and networks that elevate and uphold you. Ditch harmful connections that breed cynicism and body-disgracing. Encircle yourself with people who esteem you for what your identity is, not exactly what you look like.

PRACTICE POSITIVE CONFIRMATION

Negative self-talk can be impeding to your confidence. Battle those internal pundits by rehearsing positive assertions. Help yourself everyday to remember your value, abilities, and uniqueness. Embrace the mantra that your worth isn't attached to your appearance.

CENTER AROUND WELLBEING, NOT WEIGHT

Moving the concentration from weight to in general wellbeing is essential for feeling significantly better in your skin. Wellbeing envelops something beyond actual perspectives; it additionally incorporates mental and close to home prosperity. Focus on exercises that support your spirit and upgrade your general health.

ENTERTAIN YOURSELF

Web-based entertainment can be a situation with two sides with regards to self-perception. Recall that most photographs online are arranged and sifted, not a precise portrayal of the real world. Oppose contrasting yourself with these glorified pictures. All things being equal, develop self-empathy and advise yourself that everybody has their battles.

TAKE PART IN BODY-POSITIVE MEDIA UTILIZATION

Pick media that advances body inspiration and variety. Encircle yourself with content that features an extensive variety of body shapes and sizes. This openness can assist with reshaping your view of magnificence and challenge thin excellence guidelines.

Put forth Practical Objectives

Laying out unreasonable body objectives can prompt dissatisfaction and frustration. All things being equal, center around defining reachable and solid objectives that further develop your general prosperity as opposed to exclusively zeroing in on appearance.

Look for Proficient Assistance IF Vital

Assuming that you battle with self-perception issues notwithstanding your earnest attempts, looking for proficient assistance can be advantageous. Conversing with an advisor or guide gaining practical experience in self-perception and confidence can give significant bits of knowledge and backing.

Mirroring your external excellence:

Inward excellence rehearses that think about your external magnificence
I have as of late begun training ladies on different viewpoints that have assisted me with improving as a, more satisfied and more joyful individual and I felt like it was something that would really merit imparting to you as well. I have assembled what I accept makes all the difference for keeping an overall solid and blissful way of life which thus assists how we with searching externally as well.

• **Reflecting your outer beauty**

I have assembled what I accept makes all the difference for keeping an overall solid and blissful way of life which thus assists how we with searching externally as well.

These work for me so I chose to impart these practices to you. Trust you partake in the short perused.

Uplifting outlook: When you deal with your inward magnificence, you foster an inspirational perspective that considers your external excellence. You are bound to grin, ooze certainty, and have a more cheery disposition. This positive energy is infectious and alluring, making you more congenial and amiable.

Stress the executives: Dealing with your inward magnificence includes dealing with your feelings of anxiety, which can fundamentally affect your external excellence. Stress can cause an extensive variety of skin issues, like skin break out, dermatitis, and untimely maturing. By overseeing pressure through exercises like reflection, exercise, and taking care of oneself, you can keep up with solid, brilliant skin.

Certainty: Dealing with your internal excellence by rehearsing taking care of oneself, self esteem, and dressing great can assist with helping your certainty. At the point when you feel certain within, it reflects in your stance, looks, and non-verbal communication, which eventually upgrades your external excellence. So spruce up in your #1 outfits and on the off chance that cosmetics likewise helps your certainty, put some on and you'll quickly see a lift in your certainty since when you look great you feel better and spikes certainty in a split second.

Sound Way of life: Dealing with your inward excellence by embracing a solid way of life like customary activity, adjusted diet, and great rest can assist you with keeping up with great physical and psychological wellness. A solid body and brain reflect in your external magnificence through shining skin, shimmering eyes, and a fit physical make-up.

Graciousness: Being caring and sympathetic towards others is an impression of your internal excellence. It can assist you with emanating positive energy and establish an inviting climate, which upgrades your external magnificence.

Realness: Embracing your actual self and being valid is an impression of your internal excellence. It assists you with feeling OK with just being yourself, which thus, reflects in your external magnificence. At the point when you are consistent with yourself, you ooze a specific degree of certainty and balance that adds to your general magnificence.

Decreased pressure and a positive outlook : This can prompt better skin: When you deal with your emotional well-being, it can assist with diminishing pressure and advance a positive mentality. This can prompt better looking skin since pressure can cause skin inflammation, wrinkles, and other skin issues.

Better sustenance : Sustenance can upgrade your composition: Eating a decent eating regimen with a lot of organic products, vegetables, and sound fats can support your body from the back to front. This can prompt a more clear and more brilliant composition.

Normal activity: Ordinary activity can support your general appearance: Exercise can assist with further developing blood stream and oxygenation, which can prompt a seriously sparkling composition. Furthermore, standard activity can assist with further developing muscle tone, which can assist you with looking more fit and conditioned.

Taking care of oneself propensities : Its vital to rehearse taking care of oneself as it can prompt a more sure disposition: Dealing with yourself, whether it be through standard activity, a loosening up shower, or getting some margin for your side interests, can assist with supporting your certainty and confidence. This can assist you with projecting a more sure and certain disposition, which can improve your general appearance.

Rehearsing appreciation and thoughtfulness: This is critical abd something I resound with on a more profound level, it has the power that transmits energy: When you practice appreciation and benevolence, it can assist you with developing a more certain and hopeful point of view. This inspiration can emanate outwards and make you more alluring to other people. Furthermore, being benevolent to others can assist you with feeling more associated and satisfied, which can assist you with feeling more sure and blissful in your own skin.

Self esteem: When you deal with your internal magnificence, you foster an identity love and self-acknowledgment. This converts into a more significant level of fearlessness, which is a critical figure external magnificence. At the point when you love yourself, you are bound to deal with your appearance, dress such that encourages you, and conduct yourself with beauty and balance.

Conclusion: Your path to timeless beauty

As we close the pages of "New Cosmetic Beauty Skincare Guide," I want to extend a heartfelt thank you for embarking on this journey with me. It's been a delightful exploration of skincare, beauty rituals, and the diverse beauty that makes you, you. I hope you've found inspiration, learned a few tricks, and most importantly, discovered the joy in celebrating your unique radiance.

As you stand at the end of this guide, remember:

- **Final Thoughts and Encouragement:**

Your skin is your canvas, and it deserves all the love. Treat it with kindness, not just through products but with positive thoughts and healthy choices.

Change is beautiful. Your skin evolves, so let your routine evolve with it. It's a journey, not a destination.

You're a masterpiece in progress. Every experiment with makeup or skincare is another stroke on your canvas. Don't be afraid to express yourself boldly.

Your kind of beautiful is the best kind. Embrace your uniqueness, and let it shine in every aspect of your routine.

Resources for Ongoing Support:

Stay connected with the beauty community. Dive into forums, social media groups, and follow influencers for ongoing inspiration and shared experiences.
Seek advice from skincare experts or makeup artists for that personal touch tailored to your needs.
Keep exploring. Beauty is a dynamic world. Stay updated on trends and new products to keep your routine fresh and exciting.
This isn't the end; it's just a checkpoint in your beauty journey. May your reflection in the mirror always bring a smile, and may your beauty continue to evolve and unfold like a cherished story.

With heartfelt thanks and warm wishes,
[Jennifer D. Elvis]
[Author of "New Cosmetic Beauty Skincare Guide"]

Review page

Dear Readers,,

I hope this message finds you well! I'm reaching out to express my sincere gratitude for choosing to explore "New Cosmetic Beauty Skincare Guide." Your support means the world to me, and I genuinely hope the book has been a valuable resource in your skincare and beauty journey.

If you've enjoyed the guide and found it helpful, I would be immensely grateful if you could take a moment to share your thoughts with others. Your review can make a significant impact on helping more readers discover the insights and tips within the book.

To leave a review, simply visit Platform where the book is available for purchase and find "New Cosmetic Beauty Skincare Guide." Your honest feedback, whether it's a few words or a detailed review, is highly appreciated.

Thank you for being part of this journey, and I look forward to hearing your thoughts.Feel free to customize the text as needed, and provide a direct link to the platform where readers can leave their reviews. Personalizing the message and expressing gratitude can encourage readers to share their feedback.

Warm regards,

Jennifer D. Elvis
Author, "New Cosmetic Beauty Skincare Guide"